No. 1779
$18.95

MAKE YOUR OWN
EXERCISE EQUIPMENT

JACK WILEY

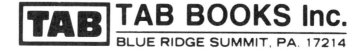

TAB BOOKS Inc.
BLUE RIDGE SUMMIT, PA. 17214

Other TAB Books by the Author

No. 1242 *How to Fix Up an Old Boat on a Small Budget*
No. 1297 *The Fiberglass Repair & Construction Handbook*
No. 1639 *Wood Carving with Projects*
No. 1669 *The Kite Building & Kite Flying Handbook with 42 Kite Plans*

FIRST EDITION

FIRST PRINTING

Library of Congress Cataloging in Publication Data

Wiley, Jack.
Make your own exercise equipment.

Includes index.
1. Exercise—Equipment and supplies—Design and
construction. I. Title.
GV543.W55 1984   688.7   84-16428
ISBN 0-8306-0779-X
ISBN 0-8306-1779-5 (pbk.)

Cover illustration courtesy of Larry Selman.

Contents

Acknowledgments

ALTHOUGH MUCH OF THE MATERIAL IN THIS BOOK comes from my own experiences with exercise equipment, doing exercise physiology research, teaching, and directing exercise programs at YMCAs and universities, hundreds of other people through the years have shared their knowledge and ideas with me. It is impossible to acknowledge all the help given. To the many people who freely shared their ideas, I want to extend a sincere thanks. I would like to extend a special thanks to the person who most helped me in my quest for knowledge about exercise and physical fitness—Dr. Thomas K. Cureton, world-famous physical fitness authority, my Ph.D. sponsor at the University of Illinois. I never ceased to be amazed by the number of people today who claim to have discovered the principles and concepts of physical fitness that Dr. Cureton was telling the world about so many years ago.

Introduction

THERE ARE MANY PLACES AVAILABLE TODAY THAT provide exercising equipment, including schools, recreation departments, organizations such as the YMCA, and commercial gyms and health clubs. Nevertheless, many people find it much more convenient to exercise at home. No time is lost commuting to an exercise area, and you have privacy. While almost every type of imaginable exercise equipment is manufactured, most of this equipment is expensive. An alternative is to make your own exercise equipment, as detailed in this book. In this way, you can set up a home exercise area or gym for a modest sum of money.

There has long been a need for a complete book on how to make and use home exercise equipment. I first started building equipment—horizontal and parallel bars—when I was in the sixth or seventh grade and interested in gymnastics. For these first projects, I had considerable adult help, but later on I constructed many pieces of exercise equipment on my own, including barbells and dumbbells, weight training benches, bicycle ergometers (stationary resistance pedal cycles), trampolines, pulley and weight training machines and devices, rings, trapeze bars, and unicycles of every description.

My early interest was mainly in gymnastics and circus skills. I once had the equivalent of a complete backyard circus at our house. Later I became interested in exercise for health and physical fitness purposes. This interest led to a Ph.D. in exercise physiology from the University of Illinois. While working on my Ph.D., I designed and constructed numerous pieces of exercise equipment, including bicycle ergometers for sitting, supine exercise, and physical fitness testing. I have also directed physical fitness programs at a YMCA and taught and done research at the University of South Alabama, the University of Illinois, and the University of California at Santa Barbara.

I have long been amazed at how expensive some items of exercise equipment are in comparison to how easy and inexpensive it is to make them. I have also found that used, broken down, and damaged exercise equipment is frequently available at low cost. Much of this equipment can easily and inexpensively be put back into use.

Some items of exercise equipment can also be purchased new for reasonable prices. It is often most practical to purchase some new items to go along with the equipment that you make and the used equipment that you buy.

Before constructing home exercise equipment or setting up home exercise areas or gyms, it is extremely important to have a basic understanding of what exercise is all about. The market is flooded with exercise equipment that doesn't work. It may make the manufacturers wealthy, but it does little or nothing for your physical fitness and may even be harmful.

It is important to know what exercise equipment is useful for your specific exercise needs. In this book, considerable space is devoted to the information you need to decide what exercise equipment can be beneficial to you. With or without equipment, useful exercise involves physical work. Machines can help you perform exercises not possible without them and make the exercise workloads more precise. Nevertheless, the equipment, if it has any value, does not do the work for you.

The attempt here is to be practical. Whenever possible, construction is simplified. In some cases, the equipment can be made from a choice of materials. A frame for a weight bench, for example, can be made from wood or metal. You can take advantage of available tools and materials and your own shop-working skills.

I have assumed that you have some experience working with tools and common materials. If not, I suggest that you take a course in wood or metal shop at an adult education program. Perhaps you will even be able to make a class project of some of the exercise equipment detailed in this book.

You will need tools and equipment. In some cases, you may want to do part of the construction work and have the rest done for you, such as cutting and shaping metal components yourself and then having the brazing and welding done for you at a commercial shop.

This book details not only how to make exercise equipment, but also gives ideas for setting up home gyms and exercise areas, including indoor and outdoor stations. It also covers exercising that can be done away from your home, such as running and bicycling. Bicycles are important pieces of exercise equipment, and Chapter 8 covers this important subject.

Although exercising in the privacy of your own home has many advantages, it also has the disadvantage of leaving you on your own. You don't have an instructor, trainer, or coach to guide you. For this reason, I have also included information about exercising in general and home exercise programs.

Chapter 1

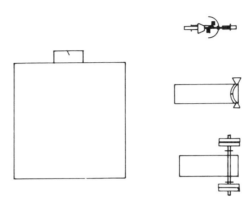

Making Your Equipment

JUMP ROPES, ISOMETRIC ROPE AND CHAIN PULL SETS, chest pull exercisers, dumbbells, barbells, sit-up platforms, weight-training press benches, exercise mats, horizontal bars, parallel bars, wall bars, horizontal ladders, balance beams, weight training devices and machines, pulley machines, and exercise pedal cycles can all be constructed at modest cost from a variety of readily available materials (Fig. 1-1). This equipment is ideal for home exercise, and it can be constructed for either indoor or outdoor use. Some of the equipment is portable; other pieces are set in the ground or attached to floors, walls, or ceilings. You can make one or two items, or you can set up a complete home workout area or gym in your backyard, patio, garage, basement, recreation room, spare room, or corner of your bedroom.

SAVE MONEY

Perhaps the most important reason for making your own exercise equipment is to save money. While a large variety of exercise equipment is now on the market and readily available, this equipment tends to be expensive. By making your own equipment and/or purchasing used, broken down, or damaged equipment and reconditioning it, you can save a considerable amount of money. By doing your own construction work, you save money not only by providing your own labor, but also by being able to purchase materials and supplies at the lowest possible prices.

The amount of money that you can save depends on many factors, including the particular piece of equipment, your ability to find and purchase required materials at the lowest possible prices, the tools and equipment you have available, and your ability.

CHALLENGE AND SATISFACTION

Many do-it-yourselfers gain considerable satisfaction from building things. Making your own exercise equipment can be challenging at all levels of skill. Some items of equipment are easy to construct and they make ideal projects for beginners. Other projects are more difficult, and some will provide a challenge even for experienced shop workers.

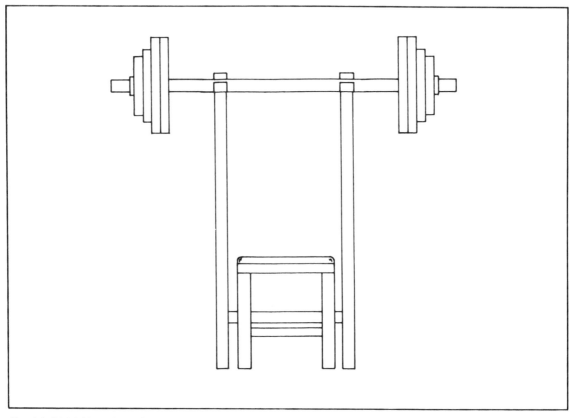

Fig. 1-1. Weight bench, rack, and barbell.

You might even want to go on to design and construct equipment to your specific requirements. For some people, making the equipment is the most important factor, others are mainly interested in having the equipment for doing exercises, and still others derive satisfaction from both making and using the equipment.

GET EXACTLY THE EQUIPMENT YOU WANT

When you make your own equipment, you can customize it to your size and requirements. You can make the equipment to fit available space. You can make portable, mounted, or permanent "built-in" equipment. To do all this, of course, requires that you have the necessary tools, materials, and skills, as detailed in this book, but when you purchase manufactured exercise equipment, you have only a limited choice— especially in the case of low-priced equipment.

WHEN TO BUILD AND WHEN TO BUY

The decision of when to build and when to buy exercise equipment is not always an easy one. If you build things all the time, you will probably have a good idea of how much time the construction of a particular piece of exercise equipment will take and how much the materials will cost. A less-experienced person will have more trouble doing this, however, and the tendency is often to underestimate both the cost and the time it will take.

In the case of a piece of manufactured exercise equipment, you will need to consider a number of factors. First, how will your finished project compare with the manufactured equivalent? Will it be of equal quality? Will it have the same appearance as the manufactured product, or at least a satisfactory appearance? And perhaps most important, will the item you make serve the same function as the manufactured equipment?

Second, how will the cost of the equipment that you make compare with that of a manufactured equivalent? If you can make the item for a few dollars and the manufactured equivalent costs a hundred dollars, then the decision to make your own should be obvious provided that you can make the piece of equipment in a reasonable amount of time. As the cost of making your own approaches that of the manufactured equivalent, the decision becomes more difficult.

Also, you will want to consider used manufactured equipment. Where I live, used weight-training benches, with weight stands that sell for from about $60 to $100 new, are often available at thrift stores and garage sales—used but in satisfactory condition—for $25 or less. Before making your own, you will probably want to be certain that you can do the job for less than you can buy a used manufactured equivalent.

Third, you will probably want to consider the time element for making your own. Is it still practical when you consider how long the construction will take?

In most cases, it is best to buy some equipment new, buy some used, and make the rest yourself.

SKILLS, TOOLS, AND MATERIALS

Before undertaking an exercise-equipment construction project, it is important to consider your skills, the tools you have, and the materials that are available. If you have the necessary skills and tools to build items of similar difficulty from similar materials, you should not have much difficulty making the exercise equipment detailed in this book. For example, making a dog house from wood is similar to making a weight-training bench from wood. This book details how to make the weight-training bench, and provided you have the skills and tools to make a dog house, you should have no difficulty.

The tools and materials required for making your own exercise equipment are detailed in Chapter 3. If you are a do-it-yourselfer, you probably have many of the tools already. A few basic tools will serve for making many of the projects, but some will require more elaborate tools and equipment, such as for brazing and welding. You can do part of the construction work yourself, however, and then farm out the jobs that you don't have the skill and/or equipment to do to a commercial shop.

PLANNING EQUIPMENT AND EXERCISE AREAS

You will need to decide what exercise equipment you want to make and/or buy, where you are going to put it and use it, and how you are going to arrange it. If you have very limited space, you may want to stick to portable equipment. You can move the equipment from place to place and out of the way for storage when you are not using it. In this way, the same area can also be used for other purposes besides exercising.

It is generally much more convenient, however, to have an area where you can leave the exercise equipment set up all the time, ready to use. After you finish your program, you don't have to put the equipment away. This might not seem very important, but I have found that many people quit exercise programs because it is just too inconvenient and time-consuming to set up and put away exercise equipment.

Indoor exercise areas can be set up in the corner of a room or a garage, or you can use a larger area—perhaps even setting up a complete home exercise gym. In any case, you will want to make the best use possible of whatever space you have available. Some equipment is freestanding in the sense that it is not attached to the floor, walls, or ceiling. Other equipment is mounted, more or less permanently, so that it can be easily set up and removed. Freestanding equipment has the advantage of not requiring fasteners in floors, walls, and ceilings for mounting brackets and other attachments. Mounted equipment often requires drilling holes for fasteners and making other modifications to floors, walls, ceilings, and other parts of a house, garage, or other structure.

Before setting up an indoor exercise area, you might first want to make improvements in the building itself, such as paneling or repaneling the walls, adding carpet to the floor, painting, etc.

Figure 1-2 shows a possible arrangement for

3

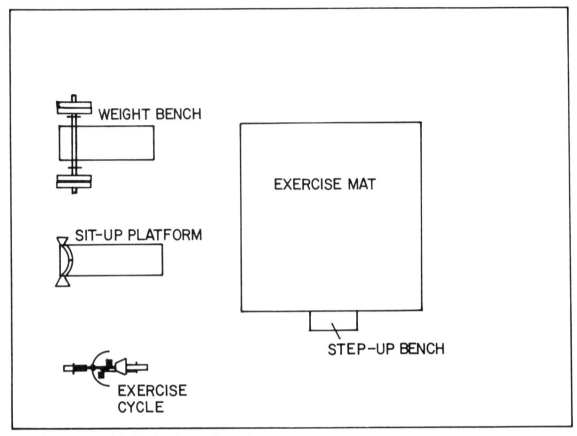

Fig. 1-2. Arrangement for freestanding equipment.

an exercise area using freestanding equipment. Arrangements using both freestanding and mounted equipment are shown in Figures 1-3 and 1-4. Before designing your own exercise area, you will, of course, need to decide what exercise equipment you want.

Portable and freestanding exercise equipment can often also be used outdoors. Many items of exercise equipment, however, will need to be stored inside when you are not using them. Another possibility is to set up outdoor equipment with posts set in the ground in cement. These items can be combined with portable and freestanding equipment.

Figures 1-5 and 1-6 show possible arrangements for outdoor exercise areas. The items of equipment can be used as stations for circuit training. For example, you run around the block, then do a set number of sit-ups using the inclined platform, then another run around the block, then a set number of chin-ups using the horizontal bar, and so on.

For both indoor and outdoor exercise areas, it's important to make a careful assessment of your exercise needs so that you will have the right equipment. The equipment should then be arranged so that it is convenient and safe to use.

Ventilation, lighting, and temperature control are important considerations. As a general rule, you will want to have adequate ventilation in the exercise area. Good lighting can make exercising more enjoyable, and temperature control makes exercising more comfortable.

The appearance of an exercise area can also make a difference. Color schemes of exercise areas can affect your mood. You will probably want to have the exercise area as pleasant as possible. Music in the exercise area can also add to the incentive to exercise.

Racks and storage areas for exercise equipment can help to keep the exercise area or room neat and tidy. You can construct racks for barbells and dumbbells so that you will have a place to put them when you are not using them.

A bulletin board is handy for posting exercise charts. Scales should be conveniently located for weighing. If possible, showers should be located nearby.

Because it is difficult to know exactly what equipment will be useful to you when you first start a home exercise program, I suggest that you start out with a minimum amount of equipment and add to this as a need develops.

PLANS AND INSTRUCTIONS

Plans and instructions for making a variety of exercise equipment are detailed in this book.

Chapter 4 covers basic exercise equipment, including jump ropes, elastic and spring chest pull devices, isometric rope and chain pull devices, dumbbells and barbells, weight training benches, weight racks, sit-up platforms, step-up benches, and exercise mats.

Chapter 5 details the construction of bars and balance beams, including horizontal or chinning bars, parallel or dipping bars, wall bars, horizontal ladders, balance beams, and push-up bars.

Chapter 7 covers weight and pulley devices and machines, including a wrist roller, knee extensor and flexor device, lever bench-press machine, lever-squat machine, single- and double-handle pulley machines, leg extension pulley machine, and inclined board with movable pulley platform device.

Chapter 8 covers regular bicycles—buying, maintaining, repairing, and reconditioning—and Chapter 9 covers stationary exercise pedal cycles, including how to build your own.

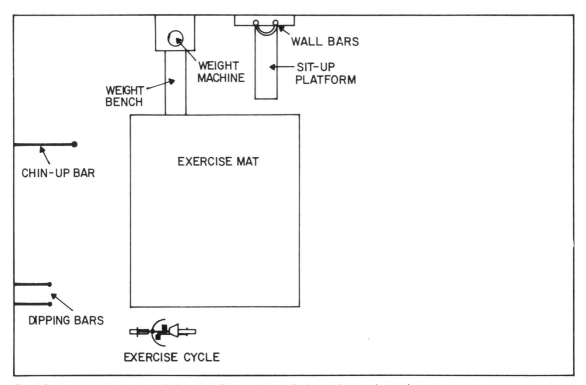

Fig. 1-3. Arrangement using both freestanding and mounted exercise equipment.

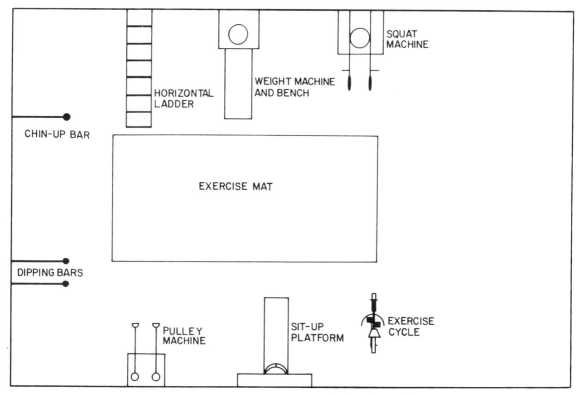

Fig. 1-4. Alternate arrangement using both freestanding and mounted equipment.

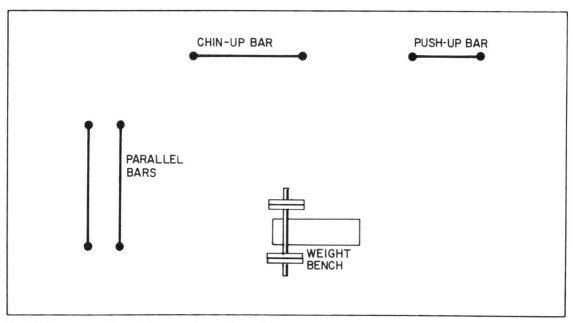

Fig. 1-5. Arrangement for outdoor exercise equipment.

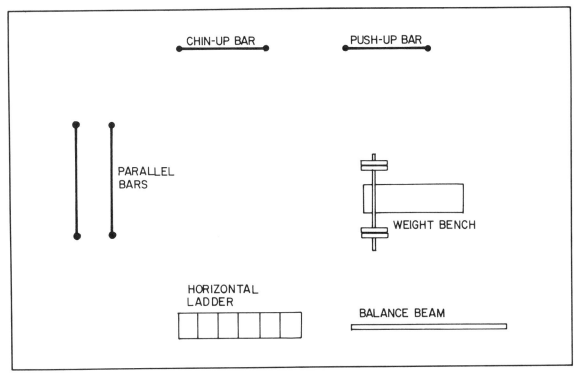

Fig. 1-6. Alternate arrangement for outdoor exercise equipment.

EXERCISE EQUIPMENT

Before going on to the actual construction of exercise equipment, consider what exercise equipment is and what it isn't. First, you can do physical fitness exercise without special equipment or with very little equipment. You can run, for example, without special equipment (but good running shoes can be a big help).

A distinction should be made between exercise equipment that has proven value and items that have no proven value or that are harmful. We are flooded with commercials for exercise equipment with fantastic claims for physical fitness without work or sweat, but present research indicates that there is no such thing. Effective exercise involves physical work. Too often, exercise equipment is thought of as machines that do the exercise for you, but this is not the case with equipment of proven value. Exercise equipment—including exercise machines, if they are properly designed and constructed—allow you to do more physical

work, not less, or to isolate and exercise specific muscle groups.

The human body is a linear motion machine. Some exercise devices, such as the bicycle, change this linear motion into rotary motion, which is continuous and ideal for endurance, cardiovascular exercise, and physical fitness.

It is important to understand that exercise equipment will not do anything for your physical fitness unless you use the equipment. Ideally, exercise should be controlled, graded, and progressive. When you run, for example, you can use time and distance covered to control the amount of exercise that you do. In this way, you can gradually and progressively work up to longer distances and/or faster times.

Many exercise machines also allow you to have at least some idea of the amount of work done, such as the amount of weight lifted or the number of repetitions done. This is important so that you can chart your progress and alter your routines for the greatest benefit.

Chapter 2

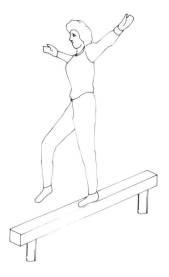

Home Exercise Programs

THERE ARE A NUMBER OF REASONS FOR HAVING home exercise programs. You might want to exercise to improve some types of physical or athletic performance or to change your body's appearance, but all of these things are closely related to good physical fitness.

Considerable confusion surrounds the term *physical fitness*. Some people think of physical fitness as being free from disability and disease, or the capacity to perform and to recover, or the increase in available energy that a person has. Three major areas of concern are the ability to perform, physique or body appearance, and organic health and efficiency.

TYPES OF EXERCISE

There are many components and attributes of physical fitness, including circulo-respiratory endurance, flexibility, muscular endurance, and strength.

Circulo-Respiratory Endurance

Circulo-respiratory endurance is being able to do exercise of a fairly high level of difficulty for long periods of time. This component of physical fitness is the most important one, at least in health terms. Endurance training such as running, jogging, bicycling, rowing, and swimming long distances in a continuous rhythmical manner are typical exercises used to improve circulo-respiratory endurance. Most physical research shows that this type of exercise should be central to any well designed physical fitness program. In fact, it is often dangerous to do some other types of exercise, especially heavy strength training, without having a high level of circulo-respiratory endurance.

While there are many ideas and concepts about how to improve circulo-respiratory endurance or fitness, most of the available research indicates that this is best done by doing some continuous rhythmical exercise for fairly long periods of time (usually a half hour or longer) three or more times a week.

Most physical fitness experts recommend that exercise programs be based on endurance. Keep this fact in mind when designing home exercise programs. There is considerable evidence that endurance exercise of the right kind and amount can improve the circulo-respiratory endurance of most people, but it should also be noted that this type of physical fitness is not permanent. If you discontinue your exercise program, you can also expect a deterioration in your circulo-respiratory endurance level.

Flexibility

Flexibility is defined as the ability to move the body parts through their full range of motion at their joints. A number of factors determine the range of motion possible in a joint, including skeletal structure, muscles, ligaments, soft tissues, and adhesions from past and present injuries. For example, the shape of bones can limit the range of motion of a joint. Muscles also limit the range of motion.

Muscles groups are arranged in pairs. The contraction of one group moves a joint to one extreme, and the contraction of the opposing group returns or moves the joint to the other extreme. From this it is apparent that if you exercise one group of muscles and not the other, flexibility problems can result from the shortening and tightening of one group of muscles. It is for this and other reasons that it is important to do flexibility or stretching exercise along with a program such as running (which tends to favor the use of certain muscle groups without exercising the opposing groups).

While opinions vary as to how best to do flexibility exercises, present research indicates that slow movements through the range of joints without bouncing actions generally give the best results with the least possibility of injury. As a general rule, bouncing and rapid movements at the extreme ranges of movement should be avoided.

Flexibility exercises, when properly done, can help to maintain and improve the range of motion of the joints, and this in turn will help to maintain full body mobility. This is an extremely important part of physical fitness and should be included along with circulo-respiratory endurance exercises.

For health and stamina, circulo-respiratory endurance and flexibility are the heart and core of a physical-fitness program.

Muscular Endurance

Muscular endurance is defined as the ability of the muscle or groups of muscles to persist in an activity or movement. This differs from circulo-respiratory endurance, in that only a specific muscle or group of muscles is involved. Jogging or running for an hour enhances circulo-respiratory endurance; how many push-ups you can do relates to muscular endurance. In the case of jogging or running, a person becomes fatigued because the body cannot supply adequate oxygen to the muscles. In the case of the push-ups, a person stops because certain muscles of the arms and shoulders become fatigued.

Muscular endurance should not be confused with *muscular strength*. Muscular strength is the maximum effort made by one contraction of a muscle or groups of muscles. Muscular endurance is the ability to repeat a strength exercise a number of times.

As a rule, muscular endurance is developed by *dynamic* or *movement exercise* by the *overload principle*, (muscles are repeatedly and regularly stimulated by a greater-than-normal exercise load and/or at a greater-than-normal rate). The same principle is used to develop strength, except that for muscular endurance the resistance or work load is usually relatively low, and the exercise is performed a number of times.

For health and stamina, muscular endurance is much less important than circulo-respiratory endurance. At least a minimum level of muscular endurance should be developed and maintained, however, along with the circulo-respiratory endurance. It is my belief that only light weights and exercises using your own body weight as resistance (such as push-ups, sit-ups, chin-ups, and dips) are required for developing adequate muscular endurance. Using heavy weights can do more harm than good, especially for older adults.

Muscular Strength

Many people confuse physical fitness with *muscular strength*. Muscular strength is the maximum effort made with one contraction. This is only one aspect of physical fitness and—provided that you have a reasonable level of muscular strength—one of the least important.

How much weight you can lift, for example, is not a meaningful test of physical fitness.

Muscular strength can be *isometric* or *static*, where the muscle develops tension without changing its length, or it can be *isotonic* or *dynamic,* where the muscle changes its length. An example of isometric or static exercise is contracting a muscles against an object that cannot be moved by the contraction. An example of an isotonic exercise is lifting a heavy weight. Both types of exercise, if carried to the extreme, can be more harmful than beneficial for typical adults (and probably for all ages).

Muscular strength is developed by maximum contractions against immovable resistances or a few repetitions against strong resistance, such as lifting a heavy weight. This differs considerably from circulatory exercise, which involves many repetitions against a slight resistance.

Weight and Body Appearance

An important part of physical fitness for many people is body weight and appearance. Weight control and exercise are also related to diet, or what we eat and don't eat, so it's important to eat a well balanced, nutritious diet if you genuinely want to see an improvement in your overall health and appearance. Consult your doctor to tailor a diet specifically for you especially if you need to lose considerable weight or suffer from any health problems.

EXERCISES AND EQUIPMENT

It is advantageous to be able to control the amount of exercise you receive. In sports, such as tennis or basketball, it is extremely difficult to control the amount of exercise or to even have a measure of how much exercise you accomplished. Of course, you can play basketball for 30 minutes each day, but the amount of exercise will probably vary greatly from day to day depending on the intensity of the game and other factors.

You have much greater control when you do an exercise like jogging or running where you can easily measure how fast you cover a certain distance. You know both the intensity and the amount of time that the exercise is continued. This allows you to progressively increase the time that you exercise and/or the intensity. You can run for a longer distance, or you can run faster. You can keep records and chart your progress. For example, you might first work up over a period of time to the point where you can jog 3 miles in 30 minutes. This can be marked on a chart. Distance equals 3 miles, and time equals 30 minutes for a certain day. This time and intensity might remain the same for three workouts a week for a period of several months. Sooner or later, you will probably want to progress to a higher level. You could keep the rate or speed of running (10 minutes per mile) the same and continue for 35 minutes, covering 3½ miles. The rate is still 10 minutes per mile. Or you could keep the 30 minute time, but jog or run faster—such as covering 3½ miles in the 30 minutes. The rate is now changed to approximately 8.6 minutes per mile.

This is considerably different from playing basketball for 30 minutes, where control of the intensity is difficult to evaluate.

Some exercises, such as chin-ups, sit-ups, dips, and push-ups, are usually thought of as exercises of number (how many we can do), but they can also be timed exercises (how many can be done in a set time).

In the case of weight training exercises, a number of variables can be controlled, including the amount of weight lifted, the number of repetitions, the speed of lifting, the number of sets done, and the time between sets. There are many different ideas about how to best achieve certain results, but many physical fitness authorities believe that for general health and physical fitness, it is best to avoid lifting heavy weights. It is my opinion that weight training has considerable use and potential as athletic training for certain sports and activities, but is of little value and can even be harmful for general physical fitness training, especially for older adults. If you do work out with weights, I suggest that you stick to light ones that you can easily lift.

It is very important to select exercise equipment for the particular type of exercise that you intend to do. A regular bicycle or stationary exercise resistance cycle is ideal for cardiovascular endurance exercise. Barbells are probably of little or no value for this purpose and might even be harmful. Most people can develop all the strength and muscular endurance that they need for a high level of general fitness by doing exercises that use their own bodies as the resistance weight, like push-ups, chin-ups, sit-ups, and so on. Even running and bicycling have an element of strength and muscular endurance involved.

Regardless of the basic type of exercise program, you will probably want to include flexibility exercises, and perhaps the best equipment for these is an exercise mat.

PROGRAMS

To gain maximum benefits from exercise, you will need to have a sound exercise program. Space does not permit coverage of specific programs here, but there are hundreds of published books that detail specific programs. For general adult fitness, I recommend programs that concentrate on cardiovascular endurance, rather than weight training. Regardless, a program makes exercising more meaningful. You have a set series of exercises to follow, and you can also keep records and chart your progress.

A number of exercise programs are now presented on television—often on educational channels—and you follow along with the exercises demonstrated.

Exercise programs are also available on video or cassette tapes that you can purchase from bookstores or, in some cases, check out from libraries.

Before starting any exercise programs, a complete medical examination is in order. Tell your doctor exactly what exercise program you have in mind, and get his approval before you start. If your doctor is fat and lazy and doesn't exercise or even believe in exercise, I suggest that you find a new doctor who exercises and believes

in exercising. Medical doctors who are endurance runners are often a good bet.

The medical examination should also include physical fitness testing to determine your present fitness level and to see if you have any adverse reactions to exercising.

It has been my experience that many people start out with a program that is beyond their present level of physical fitness. I recommend starting at a very low level and then gradually working up to higher intensities and longer durations of exercise.

You might want to make some tests and measurements and keep records of these. There are a number of simple tests based on heart rate which you can do yourself. A number of books on physical fitness detail these tests.

ELECTRONIC MONITORING

A number of electronic monitoring devices are now available for home use. Many of these devices are based on heart rate. Some have feedback to exercise cycles or other exercise devices to change the workload or resistance to keep heart rate at a desired level or to control some other factor. Electronics and computers are being used for more and more things, and I think we will see even more use of these made for exercise equipment and exercising. Some exercise equipment manufacturers have computer-controlled exercise devices on the market now, and improved designs are likely to follow. These are presently quite expensive, but prices will probably come down as production and competition for selling them increase.

No matter what program you choose, be consistent yet flexible. Tailor the program to your needs, and when it is just right for you, stick to it.

Exercise and physical fitness are lifetime habits: it's never too late to start on the road to good health.

Chapter 3

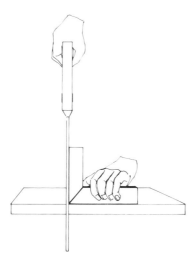

Tools, Materials, and Techniques

O NLY A FEW TOOLS, A MINIMAL WORK AREA, AND readily available inexpensive materials are required to make simple home exercise equipment. Some of the more complicated equipment requires more tools and materials that are more difficult to obtain.

In any case, take advantage of what you already have. If you have a workshop in your garage or basement, or if you do home repairs, woodworking, metalwork, or automobile repairs, you probably have some of the tools you will need for making exercise equipment. You might already have some of the construction materials such as wood, metal, fabric, old bicycle parts, and so on. Such things seem to collect in many households.

TOOLS

The right tool is extremely important for quality work. The size and nature of the particular project will dictate what tools are needed. Most constructions will require basic hand tools and a few power tools. You can select additional new or used tools as special needs arise. In some cases,

it is more economical to rent a specialized tool than to buy one. I recommend tools of at least medium quality: cheap tools are false economy—they wear out quickly or break.

Screwdrivers

The standard screwdriver (Fig. 3-1) is a basic tool designed for driving and removing screws. A screwdriver also makes a handy pry bar for removing lids from paint cans and other similar tasks, but because these jobs tend to ruin good screwdrivers by rounding the corners of the tips and distorting their shape, only old unusable screwdrivers should be used as pry bars.

Most screws have an ordinary slotted head. Screws are made in gauge sizes and each size has a specific slot width and depth. The tip of the screwdriver should fit the slot closely. Screwdrivers come with tips designed to fit specific screw-gauge sizes. Ideally, a different size screwdriver is used for each screw gauge, but it is usually possible to use a screwdriver for a screw of one gauge smaller or larger. Three or four screwdriver sizes will take care of most of the

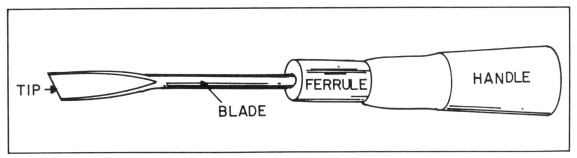

Fig. 3-1. Screwdriver.

work required for constructing exercise equipment.

A screwdriver for slotted heads should have a straight edged tip. It the corners are rounded even slightly, the tip will slip out of the screw slot.

There are also recessed-head screwdrivers. While there are a variety of screwhead types in use, the Phillips (with a cross slot) is the most common recessed type. As with standard screwdrivers, always use a Phillips screwdriver that is the correct size for the screw. Two or three sizes of Phillips screwdrivers will be adequate.

Screwdrivers come in various lengths. More leverage can generally be applied to the screw with a long screwdriver, but restricted working spaces necessitate short screwdrivers for some jobs.

Wrenches

Wrenches are used for holding and turning nuts, bolts, and various other threaded parts like pipe fittings. There are many variations with both American standard and metric openings.

Chrome vanadium steel is one of the best materials for making wrenches. It is lightweight and very strong, but it is also very expensive. Much less expensive, but still good-quality, wrenches are made of forged carbon steel and molybdenum steel. The best grades of these are dropped forged. Purchase at least medium quality wrenches.

Wrenches used on nuts and bolts should fit properly so that there is a minimum of play, yet have enough clearance to allow the wrench to slip over the nut or bolt.

An *open-end wrench* (Fig. 3-2) is a common type of fixed (nonadjustable) wrench. Often, there is a different size open end at both ends of a single handle. Generally, the smaller size openings have shorter handles than do the larger-size openings. The larger sizes require longer handles for greater leverage.

The open end or head of the wrench is often angled about 15 degrees to the centerline of the handle. This angle, and the fact that the wrench can be turned over, allows you to work in tight places. There are also right-angle, open-end wrenches and wrenches with curved handles that are useful for some jobs. The standard open-end wrenches, however, will take care of most jobs required for constructing exercise equipment.

Open-end wrenches are often available in sets of from six to ten wrenches at a savings over purchasing the wrenches individually. These

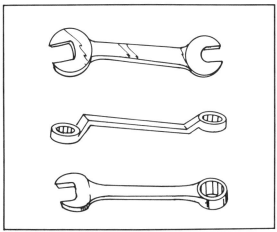

Fig. 3-2. Open-end, box, and combination open-end and box wrench.

sometimes come with a clamp that holds the wrenches together as a single unit—handy for keeping the wrench set together and organized.

A *box wrench* (Fig. 3-2) is another common type of fixed wrench. Because they are less likely to slip off a nut or bolt, they are safer to use. The box head completely surrounds the nut or bolt. This closed circle allows adequate strength with thinner walls and lets you turn nuts and bolts in tight spaces. Most box wrenches have twelve points. This makes it possible to work when only a short swing is possible. The wrench can be set over the nut or bolt at many different angles.

Box wrenches frequently have a different size head at each end. The heads are usually offset so that they can reach the heads of recessed bolts. Again, the small sizes have shorter handles than larger sizes to give the required leverage.

Box wrenches are available in sets of from six to ten wrenches in both American standard and metric sizes. It's usually less expensive to buy sets than individual wrenches.

Combination open-end and box wrenches (Fig. 3-2) are also available. These have a box on one end and an open end on the other. The openings are usually both of the same size. You can go most of the way with the open end when tightening a nut and then secure it with the box end. These wrenches often have offset handles on the box ends. Combination wrenches are convenient, but it takes twice as many to make a complete set as with box or end wrenches alone.

A variety of *socket wrenches* (Fig. 3-3) is available. A typical set consists of a variety of sockets and several types of handles, extension bars, and adapters. The sockets have six and 12 points. Extra-long sockets, called *deep sockets*, are also common. Handles include hinged, speed, ratchet, and sliding T-bars, and extension bars of various lengths are used. Universal sockets and joints allow additional socket uses, as do male and female adapters.

Socket sets usually include a variety of socket sizes in either American Standard or metric sizes (some sets now include both), and some or all of the handles, extensions, and adapters listed above. Sockets have a square opening on one end that fits the square drive lug on the handles. These come in ¼-inch, ⅜-inch,

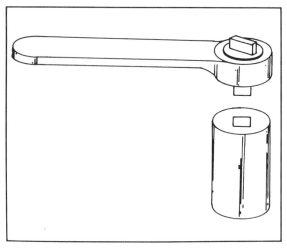

Fig. 3-3. Socket wrench.

and ½-inch sizes; this is called the *drive size*. Each socket has a second sized opening on the other end that fits the nut or bolt.

Socket wrenches, while not essential for the construction of most exercise equipment, can be helpful. A set of socket wrenches of at least medium quality is a good investment. These will do most of the jobs of open-end and box wrenches faster, easier, and more conveniently and do many jobs that are difficult or impossible with open-end and box wrenches.

Allen or hex wrenches are used to fit recessed hexagonal openings in the heads of the fasteners. While you probably won't be using these types of fasteners for the equipment that you construct, they are sometimes found on equipment that you will be repairing, adjusting, or reconditioning. Allen or hex wrenches are available individually or in sets in three basic styles: shaped like a key, L-shaped, and in a pocket knife configuration.

Torque wrenches permit the user to determine the torque being applied to the fastener. These will not be needed for the construction of most exercise equipment.

Adjustable wrenches are available in two basic types: the no longer popular *monkey wrench* (you've probably heard many jokes about this one) and the *crescent wrench*. Crescent wrenches (Fig. 3-4) are available in various sizes from about 4 inches to 24 inches in length. Longer lengths have larger jaw openings.

Whenever possible, I suggest that you use fixed and socket wrenches. There will come a time, though, when an adjustable wrench is the only one that will do a particular job, such as when you don't have any other wrench that will fit the particular nut or bolt. Adjustable wrenches are sometimes called "knuckle busters" because of their tendency to slip off the nut or bolt when improperly used. To avoid this, choose a wrench of a size suitable for the job. Adjust the wrench so that it fits the nut or bolt securely. Position the wrench so that the fixed jaw is on the side away from the pulling direction. Position the nut or bolt as far into the throat of the jaws as possible.

Pipe wrenches are available in four basic types: standard adjustable, chain, strap, and internal (Fig. 3-4). The standard adjustable-type is the most common. These are also called *straight pipe wrenches* (there is also a less common *offset* design). Pipe wrenches are useful for constructing those pieces of exercise equipment that use pipe and pipe fittings. In most cases, a standard adjustable model will suffice, but all types can be used.

Pliers

Various types of pliers are used for gripping and holding small items, cutting, stripping, and crimping. In fact, there are over a hundred different types and sizes of pliers being manufactured. It is important to select pliers carefully so that they have maximum usefulness for your particular purposes.

Slip-joint pliers (Fig. 3-5) are often considered "regular" pliers. The jaws can be positioned either for grasping small or large objects. Many types of slip-joint pliers feature a wire cutter at the base of the jaws. These are suitable for cutting soft materials such as nails and easy-to-cut wires. Slip-joint pliers, with or without wire cutters, are available in lengths from about 5 to 10 inches with various shapes of jaws.

Utility pliers (Fig. 3-6) have wide capacities and can be adjusted to a number of different positions by means of multiposition slip-joints or tongue-and-groove adjustment. They come with various lengths of handles: long handles provide considerable leverage for gripping and holding objects.

Long-nose pliers (Fig. 3-7) come in a variety

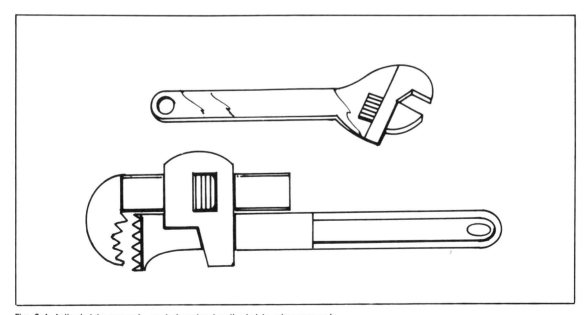

Fig. 3-4. Adjustable wrench and standard adjustable pipe wrench.

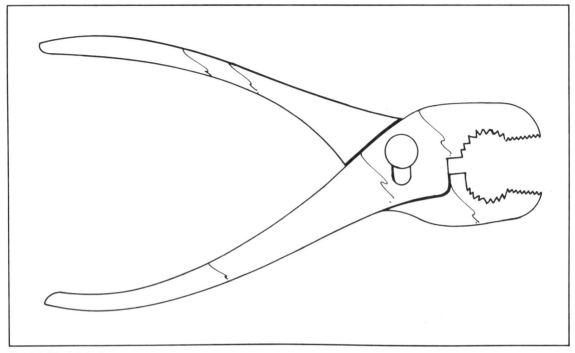

Fig. 3-5. Slip-joint pliers.

of configurations. Designs with and without side cutters are available. Long-nose pliers are used for holding and moving small objects and doing a variety of other intricate tasks. You will probably want to have one or more of these in your tool kit.

Side-cutting pliers (Fig. 3-7) are useful for holding, bending, and cutting thin materials. These are available in various lengths.

Locking pliers (Fig. 3-8) can be clampled on an object, and they will stay in place. These are available in various sizes. Follow the manufacturer's instructions for adjusting the particular brand.

Diagonal-cutting pliers (Fig. 3-9) come in various sizes and designs for light- and heavy-duty cutting. These are for cutting only and should not be used for gripping and holding objects.

End-cutting pliers (Fig. 3-9) are often called "nippers." They are available in various designs and sizes. They have a good mechanical advantage that makes them suitable for heavy-duty use.

Vises

Vises are important tools in constructing exercise equipment. The type and number of vises depend on the kind and amount of work you intend to do. A woodworking bench vise or a work table with a vise arrangement built in provides a convenient method for clamping and holding a variety of wood sizes and shapes. Machinists; utility bench, and pipe vises find a variety of uses in mechanical and metal work. Some vises are bolted to the workbench, others, generally lighter, have clamp-on bases so that they can be attached to any convenient bench or table.

Clamps

Many different *clamps* are available that are useful for holding work together. These are used for fluing and a variety of other tasks. A common and extremely useful type is the *C-clamp*. These come in a variety of sizes. They are available for light-, medium-, and heavy-duty use.

16

You may also find other clamps, such as *bar* and *pipe clamps* with wide openings, useful for some exercise equipment construction tasks.

Hammers

A variety of kinds and sizes of hammers are available, each intended for a specific range of uses. Using them for other purposes can damage the hammer or the materials you are working on and may present a safety hazard.

Claw hammers (Fig. 3-10) are frequently called nail or carpenter's hammers. Their purpose is to drive and pull or draw out nails. They are available with either curved or straight claws. The nail driving face of the hammer might be flat, slightly rounded, or even convex. The plain flat face is recommended as a general purpose hammer. Some hammers have a wooden handle attached to the steel head. Others have a steel handle that is one piece with the head and a rubber or plastic grip. Fiberglass handles are also available. While claw hammers come in a variety of weights, one with a 16-ounce head is recommended for general use. Because a hammer is a frequently used tool, I suggest that you buy one or more of at least medium quality.

Ball peen hammers (Fig. 3-10) are available with wood, steel, and fiberglass handles. The ball peen end can be used for striking in areas where the face will not fit. They are designed for striking punches and cold chisels, shaping and straightening metal and riveting work. They come in a variety of weights: a 12-ounce hammer is about right for general use. Other weights can be added if you need them.

Mallets (Fig. 3-10) are hammers with soft material heads. They are used in situations where a steel hammer would cause damage, such as when striking wood or plastic. Mallet faces are made from a variety of materials, including wood, plastic, rawhide, and rubber.

Other hammers that might be useful for constructing exercise equipment include *scaling* or *chipping hammers* for welding and *sledge hammers* for driving stakes and other similar tasks.

Hatchets and Axes

Hatchets and *axes* can be used for cutting, splitting, and trimming wood and might be useful for constructing some types of exercise equipment, such as wood posts for outdoor horizontal bars.

Prying Tool

A *crowbar* is a useful prying tool. These come in a variety of lengths and shapes.

Saws

Saws are available for cutting wood, metal, plastic, and other materials. Saws should be used only for their intended purposes. The selections

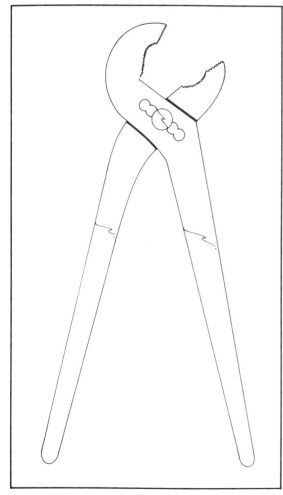

Fig. 3-6. Utility pliers.

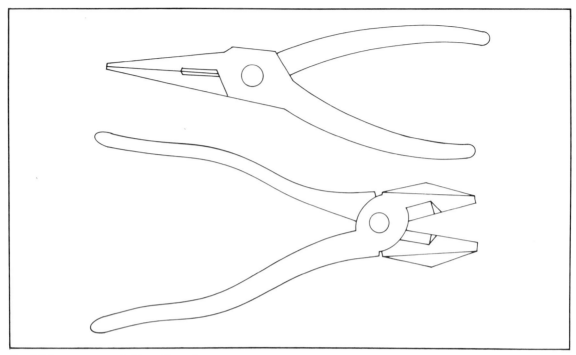

Fig. 3-7. Long-nose and side-cutting pliers.

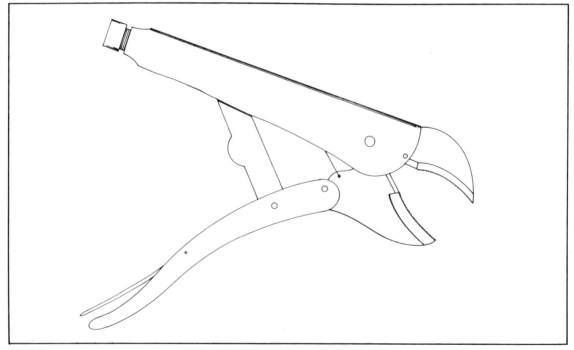

Fig. 3-8. Locking pliers.

18

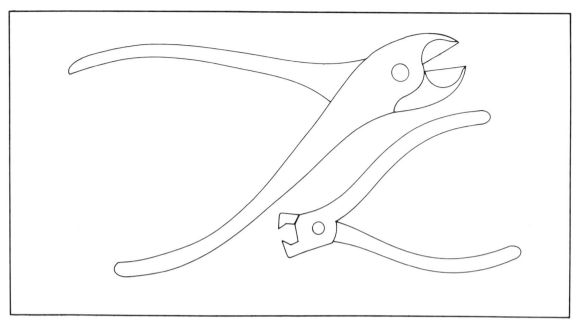

Fig. 3-9. Diagonal cutting pliers and end-cutting pliers.

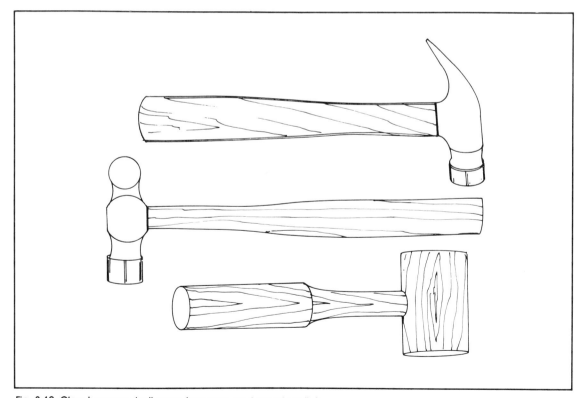

Fig. 3-10. Claw hammer, ball peen hammer, and wood mallet.

of saws will depend on the particular work you intend to do.

A variety of handsaws are available for cutting wood. Most types feature a blade with a handle at one end.

Generally speaking, you get what you pay for in saws. In addition to conventional steel blades, there are now coated-steel blades that provide a self-lubricating quality that makes cutting easier and adds rust protection.

While there are multipurpose saws for crosscutting (sawing across the grain) and ripping (cutting with the grain), these tend not to do either job very well. It is generally much better to have both a crosscut saw and a ripsaw. The difference is in the size, shape, and set of the teeth. A general purpose ripsaw might have four and one-half teeth per inch and a crosscut might have seven teeth per inch. The ripsaw teeth are set so that they cut chips. The crosscut teeth are set so that they cut two parallel grooves.

Other useful handsaws for cutting wood include the *coping* saw, *keyhole* saw, *compass* saw, *backsaw*, and *dovetail* saw.

A coping saw is used to cut curves and make interior cutouts (Fig. 3-11). Blades are available for cutting wood, plastic, and soft metals.

Keyhole saws are useful for making cutouts. A compass saw is similar to a keyhole saw, but with a wider blade. The compass saw is designed for sawing curves. A single handle often fits interchangeable blades for keyhole and compass saws.

The backsaw is designed so that perfectly straight cuts can be made across the wood cleanly without splintering. The backsaw is useful when accurate cutting is required.

A dovetail saw is designed for the fine cutting required in making dovetails. It is similar to a backsaw, except that it has a thinner blade. This saw is useful when very accurate cutting without chipping and burring is desired.

A variety of portable power saws are available for cutting wood. If you do any quantity of work, you will probably want to add one or more of these to your tool collection.

Portable *saber saws* are useful not only for cutting wood, but also, with special blades, plastics and soft metals. I suggest at least a medium quality saw. I have found that variable

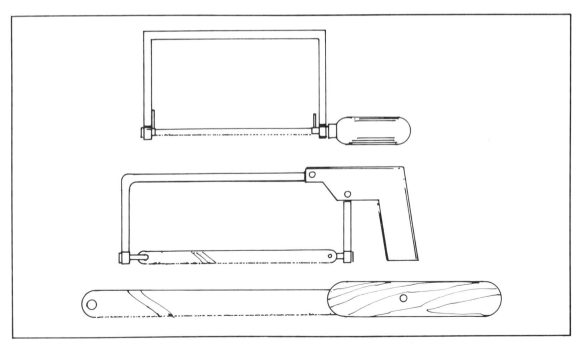

Fig. 3-11. Coping saw, hacksaw with traditional frame, and hacksaw with file-type handle.

speed control is a handy feature. Follow the manufacturer's instructions regarding what blade to use for a particular cutting job.

Portable *circular saws* are useful for cutting wood; for general use, a portable circular saw with a 7¼-inch blade works well. As with all power tools, the saw should have a blade guard and other necessary safety features. Safety precautions should be observed when using and storing the saw.

Reciprocating saws and *chain saws* are other saws that may be found useful for cutting wood when making exercise equipment.

If you do a large amount of woodwork, you may want to invest in one or more stationary power saws. The *table saw, radial arm saw, band saw*, and *jig or scroll saw* are all useful for specific cutting tasks.

The *hacksaw* is the main handsaw used for cutting metal. Some hacksaws are designed for one fixed blade length and others are adjustable for various lengths of blades. Hacksaws are available with handsaw or *pistol-type* grips and *file grips* (Fig. 3-11), which can be used in areas where a regular hacksaw will not fit. Three basic teeth sets are available: *alternate, raker*, and *wave*. Blades come with various numbers of teeth per inch, depending on what metal is to be cut. The blades are made from several materials. The most expensive is hard tungsten. This works well for cutting hard metals. For general metal cutting, less expensive molybdenum blades will usually suffice. There are also *rod-saw* blades that fit standard hacksaw frames: tungsten-carbide particles are bonded to the rod. These work well for cutting hard metals.

A variety of power saws can be used for cutting metals. A limited amount of metal cutting can be done with a saber saw by using a special metal-cutting blade. There are also power hacksaws, but the cost of these limits their use in home shops.

Hole-Making Tools

A portable *electric drill* will make most hand braces and drills unnecessary. This is provided, of course, that you have a source of electricity or a "cordless" electric drill that operates from a battery. Tools for making holes by hand are useful at times and some people still make considerable use of them.

A *carpenter's brace* with a medium swing will serve for most general work of boring holes in wood. To go along with this, you will need an *auger bit* for each hole size you intend to drill, or an *expansion auger bit* that covers the range of hole sizes that you require. For example, one model available adjusts from ½-inch to 1½ inches; another adjusts from 1-inch to 4 inches.

Twist drills, which have a hand crank and either a handle or a breast plate, and *push drills* can be used for drilling holes in wood, plastic and, to a certain extent, in metals.

A portable electric drill is an extremely important and useful tool for constructing exercise equipment. While a ¼-inch drill with about 2000 rpm is adequate for most general work, a ⅜-inch model with 1000 rpm can be advantageous. Some drills have speed controls to keep the speed constant, and drills with a variable speed feature are useful. You can also get a reversing feature to help remove screws.

So-called "cordless' electric drills are also available. These have a battery pack located in the handle or in a separate case. Rechargable nickel-cadmium batteries are usually used.

In addition to a selection of standard bits for wood and metal, sanding, grinding, polishing, pilot hole attachments are also available.

Stationary power drill presses allow more precise drilling. Many types and sizes are available ranging from presses that hold portable electric drills to heavy-duty self-contained units. A variety of attachments are available for drill presses that make possible carving, shaping, sanding, and a variety of other jobs.

Chisels, Gouges, and Planes

A variety of chisels, gouges, and planes is on the market. *Chisels* (Fig. 3-12) come in a variety of shapes and sizes. For some jobs, especially with softer woods, they can be operated by hand pressure only. For hardwoods, soft-face hammers or mallets are often used for striking the ends of the chisel handles to force the beveled ends of the blades down into the wood.

Gouges (Fig. 3-13) are a special form of chisels with rounded and curved cutting ends.

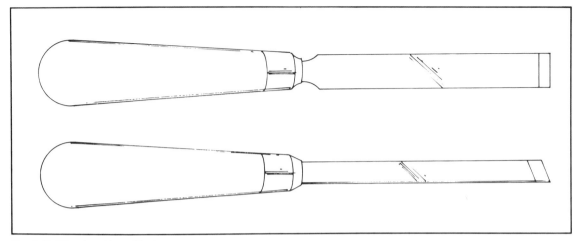

Fig. 3-12. Woodworking chisels.

They are useful for a variety of wood shaping and carving tasks, and they are available in a variety of shapes and sizes.

Planes are available (Fig. 3-14) for a variety of smoothing and shaping tasks. A *bench plane* will serve for general planing work.

Drawknives and spokeshaves (Fig. 3-15) are other useful woodworking tools.

For extensive woodworking, electric planes, routers, jointers, and shapers are good power tools to have.

Surfacing Tools, Files, and Rasps

Surfacing tools come in many shapes and sizes, such as the file-type and the plane-type (Fig. 3-16). Both flat and curved blades are available. These tools are rapidly replacing files and rasps for general woodworking.

Many shapes and sizes of files and rasps are available for woodworking, including flat, half round, round, and triangular.

Sanding Papers and Sanding Tools

Abrasive papers are frequently called "sandpaper," although sand is not actually used. The main types available are garnet paper, aluminum oxide, and silicon carbide. Abrasive papers are graded: the larger the number, the finer the grit. Most sanding is accomplished by starting with coarser grits (smaller grade numbers) and gradually working up to finer grits (larger grade numbers). Selection of abrasive papers will depend on the material to be sanded and the particular job at hand.

The abrasive paper can be held around a small block of wood. Manufactured sanding blocks with clamps for holding the abrasive paper in place are also available.

Portable power sanders are useful tools for large sanding jobs. There are three basic types: the pad sander, the disk sander, and the belt sander.

The *pad sanders* are made with orbital,

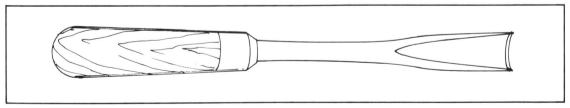

Fig. 3-13. Gouge

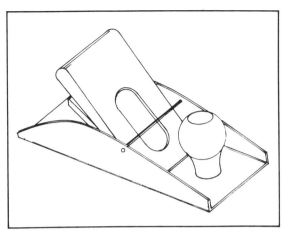

Fig. 3-14. Plane.

straight line, and combination orbital and straight line actions. Pad sanders are designed primarily for finishing and light-duty work and are used mainly for sanding wood.

Disk sanders have disks mounted at right angles to the drive spindle. They are available with disks from about 5 inches to 9 inches or larger.

Belt sanders have a belt of abrasive paper traveling over two drums. They are used for many types of sanding.

Polishing pads can be used on pad and disk sanders, and grinding attachments for metal work are available for disk sanders.

Chisels and Punches

A variety of shapes and sizes of chisels and punches (Fig. 3-17) is available for metal work. The types and sizes depend on the particular type of work to be done. Chisels can be used for cutting any metal softer than the metal from which they are made. A center punch is an important tool for marking the center of a hole that is to be drilled.

Metal Snips and Cutters

Many different snips (Fig. 3-18) are available. Most will satisfactorily cut soft and moderately hard metals. For cutting hard metals, snips with special inlaid alloy cutting edges are best. Heavy-duty cable cutters are available for cutting wire rope and steel cable: these have long handles for necessary leverage.

Metal Files

Metal files come in many different shapes, sizes, and teeth characteristics. Useful shapes include flat square, half-round, round, and triangular. Special brushes and file cards are used to remove the metal filings that tend to clog the file teeth.

Other Hand Metal Working Tools

There are many other hand powered metal working tools for making exercise equipment, including reamers, taps, dies, tube cutters, pipe

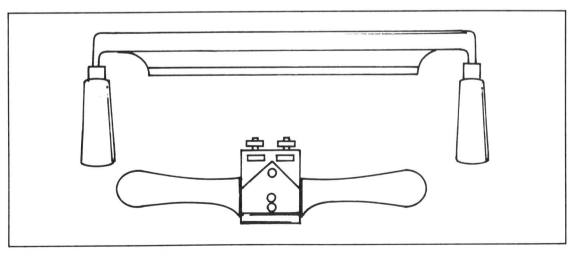

Fig. 3-15. Drawknife and spokeshave.

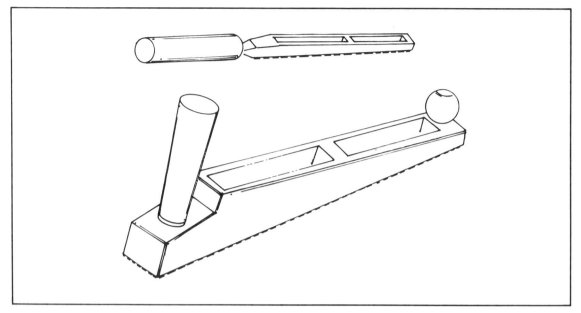

Fig. 3-16. File-type surfacing tool and plane-type surfacing tool.

cutters, pipe dies (for threading pipe), and pop rivet tools. The need for these tools will depend on the particular projects you undertake.

Power Bench Grinder and Wire Brush

A combination power bench grinder and wire brush is an extremely useful shop tool for working with metal. Grinding wheels are made from natural and manufactured abrasives. Coarse, medium, fine, and very fine (this refers to grain size) grinding wheels are available. Safety devices, including eye goggles or face shields, should always be used when power grinding or wire brushing.

When shaping metal parts, a power grinder can save considerable time over using hand files.

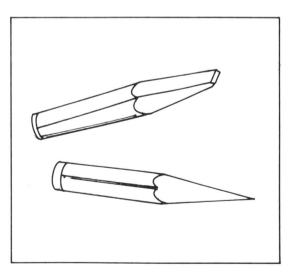

Fig. 3-17. Chisel for cutting metal and metal punch.

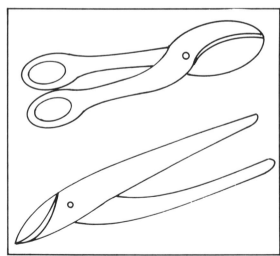

Fig. 3-18. Metal snips.

24

Measuring and Marking Tools

Tools for accurately measuring and marking are important. Two systems of measurement are in use in the United States: American Standard and the metric system. The United States is presently in the process of converting to the metric system. The systems are interconvertible (for example, 1 inch equals 25.4 millimeters), but can be confusing. If you are only familiar with one system, you will probably want to work mainly with that one and have your measuring tools in that system.

Many types and sizes of rules and tapes are available. For general use, I suggest a steel rule a yard or meter long, a zigzag folding rule, and a tape rule.

Squares are useful tools. You will probably want at least a basic *try square* to check squareness and lay out lines on the materials you are working with. A carpenter's *combination square* with 45-degree and 90-degree angles is also useful. Shop *protractors* can be used to mark and measure any angles.

A *level* is good for getting things level and vertical, such as the bar and posts for chinning bars.

Pencils, awls, and scribers are all handy marking devices, as well as pens, crayons, and chalk.

There are also many other specialized measuring tools, including calipers, micrometers, wire and rod gauges, depth and thickness gauges, and dividers. You may find some of these useful when constructing some types of exercise equipment.

Brazing and Welding Equipment

Some of the exercise equipment projects detailed in this book require brazing and welding. If you already have the skill and equipment, you will probably want to do this work yourself. If not, you can have this work done for you at a commercial shop or learn to braze and weld yourself, renting or buying your own equipment.

The two basic types of welding are gas and arc. Either or both methods are useful for joining metal parts when constructing exercise equipment.

Safety Clothing and Equipment

Safety clothing and equipment is extremely important. Always wear proper safety clothing and equipment for the work that you are doing. Goggles, shields, gloves, and dust and mist respirators are important safety devices.

Other Tools

You will need one or more sharpening stones to keep your tools sharp and in good condition. Tool boxes are good for tool storage. For shop work, a workbench with provisions for tool storage (racks, drawers, and bins), is convenient. A shop vacuum cleaner is handy.

You may also want to purchase other equipment for more specialized work, such as spray painting equipment, wood and metal lathes, and sandblasting equipment. These tools should also be useful for many other types of building and construction work in addition to making your own exercise equipment.

MATERIALS

Since construction materials are a large part of the cost of making your own exercise equipment, you can save money by shopping carefully.

In most cases, there is some waste of materials. Some of the wood, for example, ends up as scrap pieces and sawdust. You can save money by getting as much of the materials already cut to size. Whenever possible, buy in sizes that result in the least waste. While it is almost inevitable that some materials will be ruined, such as by mismeasurement or accidental splitting, try to keep these mistakes to a minimum.

What You Already Have

You may already have some of the materials that you need for making exercise equipment. Make a careful inventory. Do you have any wood that might be suitable? Are there any pipe and pipe fittings that you can use? What about nails, screws, nuts and bolts, and other fasteners? You may have one or more old bicycles that can be reconditioned for exercise riding or used for making stationary exercise pedal cycles or other exercise equipment. Old bicycle parts can be used similarly.

Used Items

By purchasing used materials, you can greatly reduce the cost of constructing your own exercise equipment. In many cases, used materials will serve just about as well as new materials, provided that you select the items carefully. Look for used items in junk stores, thrift stores, surplus stores, flea markets, garage sales, and newspaper ads.

Not only stock materials such as wood and metal pipe, rod, angle iron, bars, can be found but also items that can be used for reconditioned parts, such as weight benches, bicycles, exercise pedal cycles, and so on.

New Items

Purchasing new materials is usually more expensive than buying used, but you usually have a greater choice and more possibilities of getting exactly what you need. I buy used whatever I can find for a particular piece of exercise equipment, then buy the rest new.

Typical construction materials such as wood, pipe and pipe fittings, cement (for making barbell and dumbbells and for setting posts into the ground), rope, cables, pulleys, bolts, and other fasteners can be purchased at building supply centers and hardware stores. I have found the large discount outlets offer the lowest prices.

Marine stores offer many of the items needed for pulley machines. The mail order firm, Defender Industries, Inc., 255 Main Street, P.O. Box 820, New Rochelle, NY 10801, an ideal source for pulleys, rope, wire cables, and a variety of other items used for constructing exercise equipment. They also have canvas materials and supplies and fiberglassing materials. They charge $1.00 for their 168-page catalog.

For bicycle parts, it is usually much less expensive to buy used, but for parts you can't locate used, you can buy new at bicycle shops. Mail order sources for bicycle parts include:

—Big-Wheel Ltd., 340 Holly Street, Denver, CO 80221.

—Cycl-Ology, Wheel Goods Corporation, 14524 21st Avenue North, Minneapolis, MN 55441.

—Cyclo-Pedia, 311 North Mitchell, Cadallac, MI 49601.

WORKING WITH WOOD

Each woodworking job presents a problem—how can you best use your skills and available tools and materials to accomplish the job at hand? It is difficult to be specific about this; each job is different, yet there are some basic techniques that can be learned that will help solve many woodworking problems.

If your woodworking experience is limited, a good starting point is a class in woodworking. Many adult education programs offer such classes that allow you to learn with supervision.

Best results can usually be achieved by dividing each job into small steps. Then spend some time thinking about how these steps can best be done. Try to do each step right. Don't let sloppy work get by because it can accumulate. By the same token, if you do each step, each little job, right, the result will be workmanship of which you can be proud.

Types of Wood

The kinds of wood suitable for particular jobs varies depending on required strength, ability to take fasteners, etc. In many cases, you will have a choice of woods that will work for a particular application.

Douglas fir is a wood of medium hardness that is available in many parts of the United States. This wood works well in bench frames and other similar uses. It is also used for making plywood.

A variety of pine woods can be used similarly. White and yellow pine are especially suitable for framing work.

Redwood can be used in posts for outdoor exercise equipment. Redwood is highly resistant to rot, but it tends to be brittle and have a low resistance to shock.

Some items of equipment, such as wall bars and handles for pulley machines, require hardwoods, such as oak. Dowels shaped from hardwoods are readily available from building supply centers.

Plywood is required for a number of the exercise equipment projects detailed in this book. Plywood is made of veneers laminated together. Douglas fir is a popular wood for making plywood, but other woods, like hardwoods, are also used, especially for outer faces.

Interior grades of plywood are made with a non-waterproof glue and are not recommended for use on exercise equipment, even though you may not intend to get the equipment wet. This type of plywood tends to delaminate from moisture even when painted or varnished.

Exterior grades of plywood should be used for exercise equipment. Plywood usually comes in standard 4 × 8 feet sheets, but is sometimes available in both smaller and larger sizes, such as 2 × 4 feet and 4 × 16 feet. Plywood is commonly available in ¼-inch, ⅜-inch, ½-inch and ¾-inch thicknesses. Also manufactured are ⅛-inch and 1-inch thicknesses.

Shaping Wood Parts

A fundamental woodworking skill is shaping wood parts. In some cases, you will have a *template* or measurements for the part. In other cases, you can take measurements from where the part will fit and transfer these to the wood. Often, the measurements are marked on the wood with straight lines made with a pencil or scribing tool and a straight edge or square.

In any case, a pattern correctly marked on the wood to be used is preliminary to cutting and shaping the wood to the desired size. Make certain that you use wood that is suitable for the job and use it in such a way as to keep waste to a minimum. If, for example, a certain part requires only part of a piece of wood, pattern it on the wood in such a way that the wood that remains will be of a size and shape that can be used later. This will require you to look ahead to future work, but it's usually worth the trouble since reducing waste can result in considerable savings. Remember, it's what ends up as part of the exercise equipment that counts.

Buying lumber, in turn, is an important consideration. You will want to purchase the lumber in sizes that will result in the least waste. In most cases, you will buy lumber by the *board foot*, which is 144 cubic inches of wood and is equal to a piece of wood 12 inches long, 12 inches wide, and 1 inch thick. For example, a piece of wood 2 feet long, 3 inches wide, and 2 inches thick is a board foot since it totals 144 cubic inches. In most cases, though, you will actually get less wood than this. You pay for the wood on the basis of the size it was in rough form before the milling process. This is why a 2 × 4 is actually less than 2 inches by 4 inches. Usually, about ⅛ inch to ¼ inch is removed from a board in the milling process. This ends up as sawdust, but you still are paying for it in the board foot pricing scheme.

In the case of plywood, the situation is different. Plywood is usually sold as sheets that are the full specified thickness.

In some cases, you may want to have the lumber yard saw a larger piece of wood into smaller pieces, with or without milling or surfacing the rough sawn edges. There is usually a charge for this, but it can be well worth it if you do not have the tools to do this work yourself. There might also be cases where you will want a piece of plywood cut into two or more pieces. Some lumber yards will make one or more cuts for you, but there is often a service charge for this. Also, some lumber yards will cut and sell you part of a full sheet of plywood.

Take care in laying out and marking the pattern on the wood to be used. Use a sharp pencil or fine scribe for marking.

There are many situations where you have a length of lumber of the desired width and thickness, and all that is necessary is to cut it the correct length with square ends. First, select a suitable board. If some pieces of your lumber have more checks, cracks, or knots than others, you will want to make your selection on the basis of where the particular piece of wood is going to be used.

Since lumber frequently has checks or cracks near the ends when it comes from the lumber yard, you may want to mark a square line near one end of the board and later saw away this section. This wastes a small amount of lumber, but it is necessary for quality work in some situations. The blade of the square is positioned firmly against the edge of the board with the outside edge of the tongue of the square lined up where the cut is to be made (Fig. 3-19).

With a sharp pencil, make a line on the board following the tongue of the square. A fine

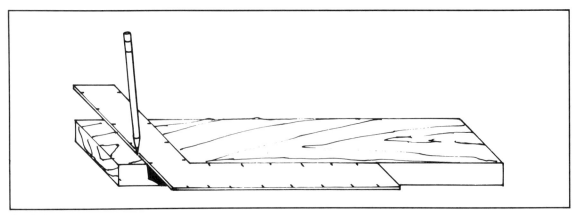

Fig. 3-19. Use of square.

line should follow as close to the edge of the square as possible. Using a suitable measuring rule, lay out the desired length from the first line along one edge of the board.

As a double check, you might want to lay out the length and make a mark a second time on the other side of the board. Use a square as described above. With the blade against the edge of the board, the tongue should line up with both marks. If it doesn't, the original end of the board was not marked off square, the edges of the board are not straight and parallel or, most likely, laying out the lengths was not done accurately. When everything looks okay, mark the line.

There are three systems to follow when the final cut is to be made: the line will be cut away, half the line will be cut away, or the cut will be made at the outside edge of the line so that the line will be visable after the cut is made. In situations where a good fit is critical, the system to be used must be taken into consideration. I suggest that you select one system and then stick to it. Always cut the lines away, or half away, or leave the line. Learn to lay out and mark your work for the system you are using.

Frequently, you will need to lay out and mark widths for later cutting. Using a measuring rule, measure and mark the desired width from one edge of the board near each end and in the middle. Then place a straight edge on the board so that one edge lines up with the three marks. If the three marks do not line up, an error was made in the measuring and marking on the

board or the edge of the board is not straight. Once you have the marks lined up, use a sharp pencil to mark the line for later cutting.

An alternate method that can be used on fairly wide boards is to use a square in the same way as for laying out and marking squared off lines across a board for length cuts, as detailed above. For this to be accurate, the end of the board must be fairly wide to give adequate distance for placing the blade of the square, and the end of the board must be perfectly square.

There are situations where you will want to lay out angles. A shop protractor can be used for this or you can use a carpenters' adjusting bevel and a protractor. Use the protractor for adjusting the bevel to the desired angle. Position the handle of the bevel firmly against the edge of the board and mark along the blade.

The same methods can be used for laying out and marking lines on plywood. A large square, long measuring rule, and straight edge are handy for this. There is some danger of making an error when extending a line. An example would be when the tongue of the square does not extend far enough and you have to add to the line.

After the pattern has been marked on the wood, the next step is usually sawing it to shape. A variety of hand and power saws can be used, as detailed previously.

Crosscutting means making a straight cut across the grain of the wood. If a handsaw is used, it should have a crosscutting blade. Crosscut saws have teeth that are the shape of small knife blades, as shown in Fig. 3-20. The teeth are bent or set alternately to the right and the left. This allows the saw to cut wider than itself and keeps the saw from buckling or binding in the wood. Crosscut saws are used for cutting across the grain of wood or at slight angles to the grain of the wood, as shown in Fig. 3-21.

Fasten the board to be cut in a woodworking vise so that the line where the cut is to be made extends an inch or so beyond the vise. Long or wide boards that cannot be placed conveniently in the vise can be placed across two or more sawhorses.

Because the saw actually cuts out a narrow section of wood, which ends up as sawdust, be sure to take this into account when positioning the saw to start the cut. Begin sawing with several short strokes. Use a small square to make certain that the saw is at right angle to the wood

(Fig. 3-22). Begin cutting again and this time use long strokes. A crosscut saw is generally held at an angle of about 45 degrees to the surface of the wood, as shown in Fig. 3-23.

Stop periodically and check the angle of the saw with the square. With experience, you will probably be able to saw through the board without twisting the saw. When you are close to sawing through the board, hold the end of the part that is being cut off in your left hand and finish the cut with short easy strokes to keep the board from breaking off or splitting from its own weight. If the wood is not too wide, a miter box and a backsaw can be used to make the same cut with even greater accuracy.

A portable power circular saw with a crosscutting or general purpose blade can also be used for crosscutting the board. Even better are stationary table power saws and radial arm saws. When using power saws, follow good safety practices: dress properly for working, follow all safety instructions for the safe operation of the particular tool, and use all necessary safety devices such as blade guards and shields.

Crosscuts can also be made at angles other than 90 degrees to the top edge of the board. It takes considerable practice to do this accurately with just a handsaw. Some miter boxes can be adjusted for performing these operations with a backsaw. The blades in most power saws can be angled as desired to the wood to be cut, making these jobs simple and accurate.

A ripsaw has chisel-like teeth. Ripsaws are designed to cut with the grain of the wood, as shown in Fig. 3-24. The teeth are essentially vertical chisels that plow out tiny pieces of wood. Like crosscut saws, ripsaws also have a set to the teeth. The ripsaw teeth are cut straight across, with chisel edges rather than knife-like blades, as on crosscut saws.

In most cases, a pattern line is first marked on the wood with a pencil or by other means. This is especially important when an accurate cut is desired.

Long pieces of wood can be placed across sawhorses for cutting. Smaller pieces of wood can be clamped in a vise to hold the wood securely while sawing.

Start the saw cut by placing the cutting edge of the blade on the desired cutting line and

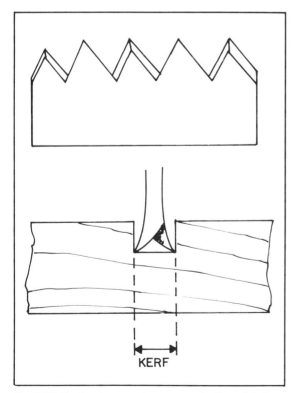

Fig. 3-20. Teeth of crosscut saw are set alternately from right to left.

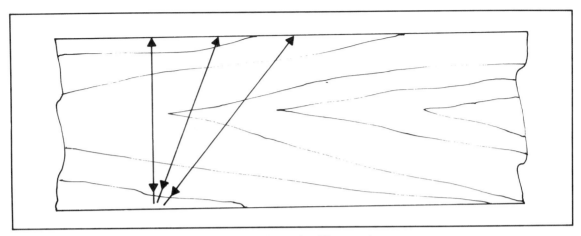

Fig. 3-21. Crosscut saws are used for cutting across the grain of the wood.

drawing the blade toward you. The saw actually removes a thin section of wood, converting it to sawdust, and this fact should be taken into account when making saw cuts. The thin section of wood that is removed, which is called the *kerf*, should be in the waste stock. Starting the cut by

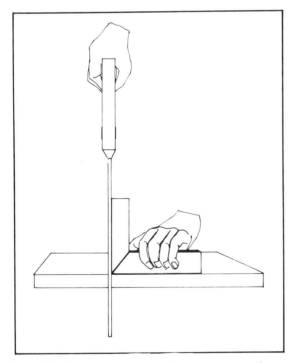

Fig. 3-22. Using a try square to check squareness of saw cutting.

drawing the blade toward you usually permits starting the cut without having the blade jump off the pattern line, as often happens when an attempt is made to start a cut by pushing the saw away from you immediately.

After starting the cut, most of the actual cutting is done when the blade is pushed away from you. A ripsaw is generally held at an angle of about 60 degrees to the surface of the wood, as shown in Fig. 3-25. In order to make certain that the cut is being made perpendicular to the surface of the wood, a square can be used to check the angle.

When sawing, watch the pattern line rather than the saw itself. If sawdust forms on the pattern line ahead of the saw cut, blow this away so that you can see the line. If the saw blade starts to go off the line, twist the handle of the saw slightly to bring the cutting edge of the blade back on the line. When ripping long boards, a wood wedge can be placed in the saw cut to keep it open and help to prevent the blade from binding. When you are about ready to saw through the wood, hold the part of the wood that is to be cut off in one hand. This will serve to prevent the wood from cracking off and damaging the wood when you saw through. Since vibration can be a problem when ripping wood, especially thin stock that is clamped in a vise, the area being sawn should be positioned close to the jaws of the vise. This will require repositioning the wood in the vise as the saw cut is being made. For example, the wood is placed so that

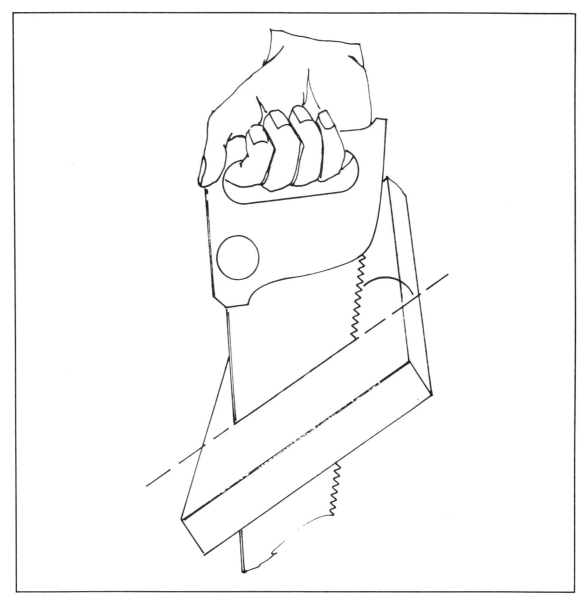

Fig. 3-23. Crosscut saw held at angle of 45 degrees to the surface of wood.

the top section of the wood extends slightly above the jaws of the vise when the cut is started. The wood is then moved up a little at a time as the sawing progresses.

Ripping can also be done with portable power circular saws, stationary table saws, and stationary radial arm saws. Use a ripping or general purpose blade.

A *coping saw,* also called a *scroll saw,* is shown in Fig. 2-20. A coping saw is useful for cutting out curved patterns in wood. A coping saw features a handle attached to a U-shaped frame. A removable blade is fastened in the frame. You can usually turn the blade to various angles in the frame. Blades, which have ripsaw type teeth, are available with various numbers of

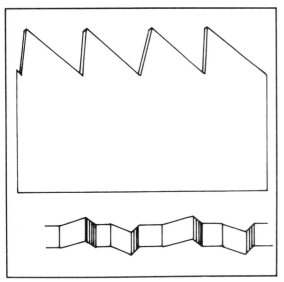

Fig. 3-24. A ripsaw with chisel-like teeth is designed to cut with the grain of the wood. The teeth of ripsaw are set alternately from right to left.

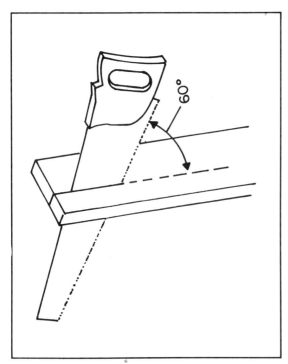

Fig. 3-25. Ripsaw held at angle of 60 degrees to surface of wood.

teeth per inch. A blade with 15 or 16 points to the inch is about right for cutting soft woods.

The wood can be clamped in a vise for cutting. The blade should be put in the saw frame so that the teeth are pointing away from the handle (Fig. 3-26). The section of the wood where you will be sawing should be positioned near the vise jaws to keep vibration to a minimum. Pattern lines are accurately marked on the wood with a pencil or by other means.

As a general rule, the cutting is done on the waste side of the pattern lines. This is important, since the saw blade actually removes a section of wood. Start the cut by drawing the blade toward you with the cutting edge placed on the desired starting point.

The actual sawing is done mainly when the blade is being pushed away from you. Try to keep the strokes even. Push the blade forward, then draw it back. The basic method for holding a coping saw is shown in Fig. 3-27. Both hands support the saw. The saw blade is generally kept vertical to the surface of the wood being cut, as shown. Move the wood in the vise as required to keep the cutting area near the jaws of the vise. Only a little downward pressure is required for cutting. Let the saw blade do the cutting. The pressure should be released on the draw strokes that return the blade to the starting position.

To make gradual curves, turn the handle of the saw to follow the pattern of the cutting line. It is important that the blade of the saw be kept at a right angle to the wood surface.

To make sharp corners, the blade is worked back and forth without any cutting pressure while the handle of the saw is turned. Twisting or bending the blade should be avoided, because you can break the blade.

For some cutting jobs, it will be necessary to turn the blade to a new angle in the saw frame. Figure 3-27 shows a typical situation where this is necessary.

To saw a cutout with a coping saw, first drill a hole inside the area of the cutout in the waste wood area. Next, remove the blade from the saw frame, insert the blade through the hole in the wood, and install the blade back in the frame, as shown in Fig. 3-28. The cutout can then be sawn. When the cutout is completed, the blade is again removed from the saw to take it

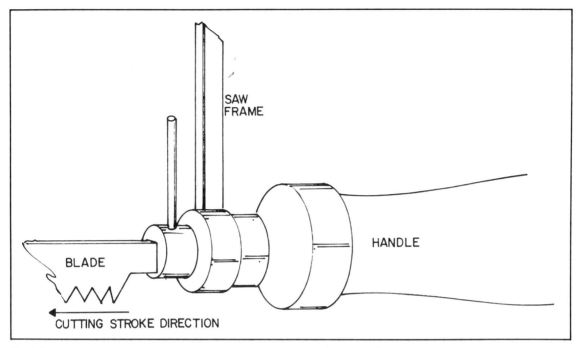

Fig. 3-26. Blade is placed in saw frame with teeth pointing away from handle.

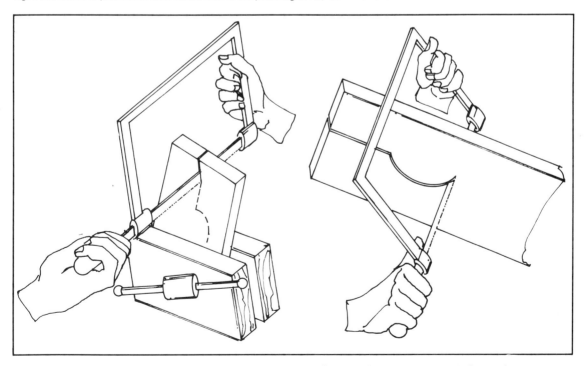

Fig. 3-27. Basic method for holding coping saw, and sawing with blade turned to new angle in saw frame.

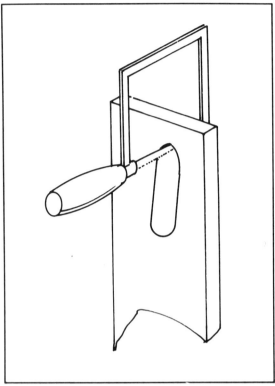

Fig. 3-28. The blade is inserted through pilot hole and installed in saw frame.

Gradual curves can be made with a compass saw by using a slight twisting action of the handle so that the blade follows the pattern line. Compass saws are limited in the amount of curve that can be sawn.

For making internal cutouts, a pilot hole is used to start the cut. While compass saws are more limited in maneuverability than are coping saws, they do offer the advantage of not requiring blade removal for internal cutouts.

Portable electric saber saws and stationary power jig saws and band saws can also be used to cut curved patterns in wood and offer faster and easier cutting than hand saws.

Sawing plywood requires special considerations. Special care must be taken to avoid chipping and splintering along the cut edge. While the sawing methods described above apply in general also to plywood, handsaws and power saws with special fine-toothed blades designed especially for plywood should be used. Even better are special carbide tipped blades. Applying a strip of masking tape over the area to

out of the cutout. To make some cutouts, it will be necessary to change the blade angle in the saw frame for various sections of the sawing.

Compass and keyhole saws can also be used for sawing curved pattern lines in wood. A typical compass saw is shown in Fig. 3-29. Compass saws typically come with several interchangeable blades for different types of jobs. The narrow points at the ends of the blades allow sawing limited curves. A keyhole saw is similar to a compass saw, only smaller. Keyhole saws are used in a similar manner to compass saws, except that their smaller sizes allow them to be used in tighter areas.

Compass and keyhole saws are usually held in one hand, as shown in Fig. 3-29. The sawing is done on the push stroke. Only slight downward pressure on the blade is required. The saw blade is usually kept vertical or nearly vertical to the surface of the wood when making straight cuts.

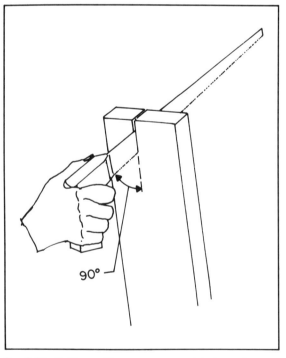

Fig. 3-29. Cutting with compass saw blade vertical to surface of wood.

be cut on both sides of the plywood, but especially the side opposite the one you are cutting from, is also helpful. Some woodworkers clamp a solid piece of scrap wood to the underside and saw through this along with the plywood.

Boring and Drilling Holes

A portable electric drill will make most hand braces and drills unnecessary. Tools for making holes by hand are useful at times, however, and some people make considerable use of them. Holes are made in exercise equipment for fasteners, as pilot holes for making cutouts, and other uses.

A carpenter's brace is a traditional tool for making holes in wood. An auger bit for each hole size you want to drill is required. A typical hole making job begins with marking the position where the hole is to be drilled. An awl or other sharp pointed device is used to start the hole. Select the correct size of auger bit and fasten it in the chuck. Make sure that it is held securely. Place the feed screw in the starting hole and begin turning the brace to start boring the hole. After the hole has been started, use a try square to make sure that the hole is being bored at right angles to the surface of the wood, assuming that this is what is desired. Resume boring until the tip of the feed screw goes through the wood. Then remove the bit, turn the board over, and finish boring the hole from the opposite side. This will help to prevent splintering.

Twist drills, which have a hand crank and either a handle or a breast plate, and push drills, which turn when pressure is applied downward on the bit, are other hand tools that can be used to make holes in wood. These drills are used in a manner similar to electric drills.

I find it much easier and more convenient to use a portable electric drill or drill press to construct exercise equipment than to use hand drills.

Ordinary twist bits from $\frac{1}{32}$-inch or less in diameter to $\frac{1}{2}$-inch or more in diameter can be used for making holes in wood. A typical drilling job using a portable electric drill is as follows:

□ Install the desired size twist bit in the chuck of the drill and secure it with the chuck key. Immediately remove the chuck key. The chuck key is frequently fastened to the cord of the drill with a special holder or plastic tape. The tool should always be unplugged when changing twist bits or other types of bits. Do not plug the drill back in until the chuck key has been removed from the chuck.

□ Make a starting hole with an awl in the position desired for the hole. Then place the point of the twist bit over the hole.

□ Hold the drill by the grip in your right hand. Start the drill and apply pressure with your right hand. Use your left hand to guide the drill. Control the drilling so that the chuck does not contact the wood when the twist drill goes through the wood. Hold the drill steady so that you do not break the twist bit. This is especially important when using small sizes of twist bits.

To drill larger holes in wood, up to about 1½ inches in diameter, spade-type bits (Fig. 3-30) are useful. To drill all the way through a piece of wood, reverse the drill after the point has gone through the wood and finish the hole from the other side.

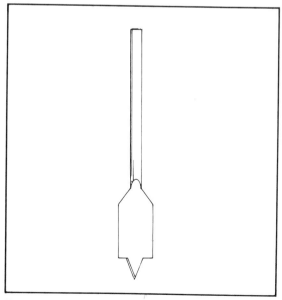

Fig. 3-30. Spade-type bit.

A hole saw (Fig. 3-31) is another useful attachment to use in power drills. These are available in sizes from about ½-inch in diameter up to 3 inches or more in diameter. Start drilling with the pilot bit, holding the drill at right angles to the surface of the wood being drilled. The drill must be kept at this angle so that the saw will cut all the way around and the hole will be vertical to the surface of the wood. To avoid splintering when the saw cuts through, clamp a piece of scrap wood underneath the piece being drilled.

One problem with the hole saw is that you are limited to set sizes, although you can use the next size smaller and then file the hole out to the desired size. An alternative is to use an adjustable *fly cutter* to make a variety of hole sizes. Use the fly cutter in a manner similar to the hole saw. Clamp a scrap piece of wood underneath the board being drilled or drill from one side to the point where the pilot bit goes through. Then, using the hole made by the pilot bit as a guide hole, finish drilling the hole from the other side.

Drill presses, which can use portable electric drills or have separate motors, are useful for more precision work.

Shaping, Planing, and Surfacing

A frequently required job is to plane the edge of a board where a saw cut has been made. While a number of types and sizes of planes can be used, a *jointer plane* works well for long boards. When

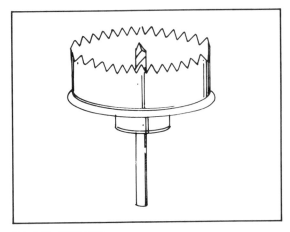

Fig. 3-31. Hole saw.

planing, use a try square to test for squareness. It is important to have the blade of the plane properly sharpened and adjusted.

Power planing and surfacing tools, especially a jointer, will make quick work of this planing job. The jointer is used to surface boards so that they can be joined together and to smooth up a rough saw cut.

Hand planes can also be used for making *chamfers*, bevels, and rounded edges on boards. Special care should be taken when planing end grain. A *block plane*, which has the blade at a more acute angle to the bottom of the plane than a jack plane, is ideal for this. Power tools, such as jointers and shapers, can also be used for these jobs.

A variety of hand tools can be used to dress and shape curved edges on wood. Rasps and files are scraping tools that have toothed surfaces. Files have teeth that are formed by long grooves set at an angle across the face of the tool. Rasps have individual teeth arranged in staggered rows. Rasps are generally used for rougher work, files are used for finer, finishing work. Both files and rasps come in various degrees of coarseness, however. This is determined by the number of teeth per square inch of scraping surface. The more teeth per square inch, the smoother. Both rasps and files are available in various shapes, including rectangular, square, triangular, half-round, and round.

The basic method for holding files and rasps is shown in Fig. 3-32. The wood to be filed should be clamped in a vise or otherwise secured. One hand is used on the handle of the tool, and the heel of the other hand rests on the front of the tool to guide and control it. The file or rasp is moved forward over the wood with a gentle forward stroke. Lift the file or rasp and move it backwards to the original starting position. Repeat the forward movement.

Files and rasps can be pushed over the wood surface in any direction with, along, or across the grain, but pushing the file or rasp against the grain of the wood should generally be avoided.

Surfacing tools are essentially modern versions of traditional rasps. Their improved scraping and cutting action is due to cutting blades on the teeth and holes all the way through the blades that allow the waste wood to pass

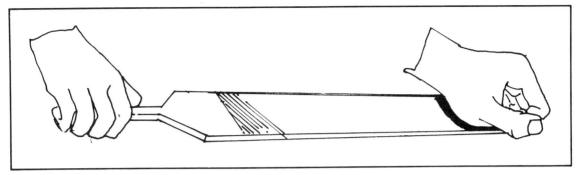

Fig. 3-32. Basic method for holding files and rasps.

through. Surfacing tools are now available in a variety of shapes and sizes, including file-types and plane-types. Surfacing tools allow you to take off a considerable amount of wood quickly.

A file-type surfacing tool is used in a manner similar to a wood rasp, except the removal of wood is generally faster and easier with the surfacing tool. The plane-type surfacing tool is held in both hands, as shown in Fig. 3-33. The hand on the rear handle is used to push the surfacing tool forward. The hand on the forward handle is used to guide and control the tool. The wood should be securely clamped in a vise. Work the blade so that you are cutting with or across the grain of the wood, but not against the grain. Apply a steady downward force on the blade of the surfacing tool as it is pushed forward. At the forward end of the forward movement, lift the tool off the wood and move it backwards to the starting position. Then repeat the forward movement again. Make as many strokes as necessary to take off the desired amount of wood or round the edge.

A *drawknife* has two handles with a cutting blade arranged so that it can be drawn toward you. Drawknives should be used with the cutting

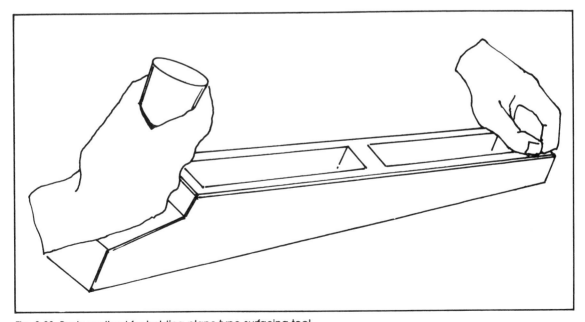

Fig. 3-33. Basic method for holding plane-type surfacing tool.

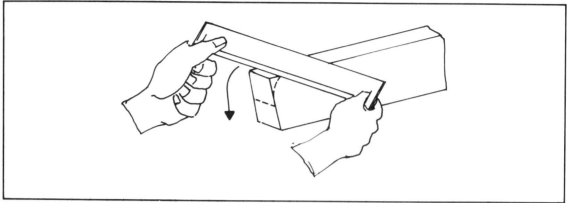

Fig. 3-34. Rounding off end of wood with drawknife.

blade moving with or across the grain, but not against it.

A drawknife can be used to round off the end of a piece of wood, as shown in Fig. 3-34. The wood is securely mounted in a vise or otherwise secured. Grip the drawknife by the handles. Place the cutting edge of the blade on the wood in the desired starting position for the first cut. The bevel of the blade should be upward. Tilt the cutting edge of the blade slightly downward and pull it toward you, making a shallow cut to remove the corner edge of the wood. Return the cutting edge of the blade to a position slightly further away from you than for the first cut. Repeat the cutting action by drawing the blade toward you. Gradually angle the cutting edge of the blade further downward as it is pulled through the wood. This will serve to round the surface of the wood.

A drawknife can also be used for contouring concave shapes that have been cut into wood with a saw or by other means. To contour the area shown with or across the grain of the wood, it will be necessary to work half of the area with the drawknife in one direction, as shown in Fig. 3-35, and reverse the wood in the vise and contour the other section.

Spokeshaves are also useful for smoothing and rounding work. The basic grip for using a spokeshave is shown in Fig. 3-36. The cutting edge of the blade is positioned at the desired starting point on the wood, and the tool is pushed forward with gentle downward pressure. When done properly, thin shavings will be lifted from the wood. By using a series of push strokes and changing the tilt of the blade, a corner edge can be effectively rounded off. Always push the tool in a direction that cuts with the grain or

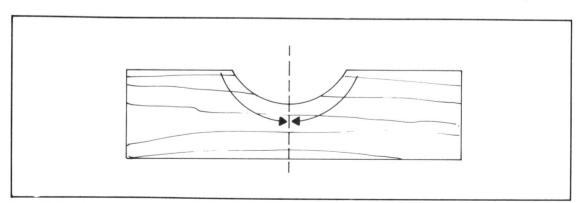

Fig. 3-35. Area is contoured with drawknife from two directions.

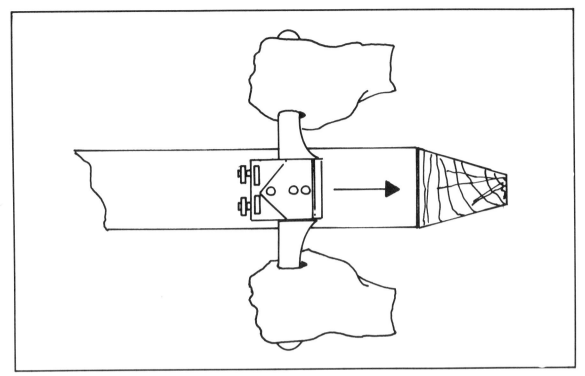

Fig. 3-36. Basic grip for using spokeshave.

across the grain of the wood, but not against the grain. When working concave areas, this often means working an area from two different directions.

Spokeshaves are useful not only for light contouring work, but also for smoothing operations. To make smoothing cuts, first adjust the spokeshave blade by means of the adjustment screws until it protrudes only slightly beyond the sole plate opening. This allows you to make a shallow cut, which is ideal for smoothing jobs.

A variety of chisels, such as those shown in Fig. 2-25, is useful for cutting, shaping, and fitting wood pieces. In many cases, the chisels can be worked by hand pressure alone. For some jobs, especially on hard woods, a wooden or other soft-face mallet can be used for striking the head of the chisel (Fig. 3-37). As a general rule, the cutting should be done with or across, but not against the grain of the wood.

Hand scraping tools, such as the *cabinet scraper,* can be used to remove irregular surfaces left by planes and other rough surfacing tools.

Joining

Joining wood pieces together and other materials to wood is an important part of the construction of many types of exercise equipment.

Two pieces of wood can be fastened together with nails, screws, bolts, wood dowels, splines, and various glues. In many cases, the joining is done both by gluing and mechanical fasteners. Gluing should only be used for joining wood pieces that are not intended to be taken apart again.

There are many alternative joints for joining two pieces of wood together, such as the *common lap joint* without a corner post (Fig. 3-38) and with a corner post (Fig. 3-39). Still another method is to use a *common scarf joint* (Fig. 3-40). This method is frequently used for joining long pieces of wood together. In many cases, the joint is held with both glue and mechanical fasteners. Still another method is to use a *butt joint* with a backing board, as shown

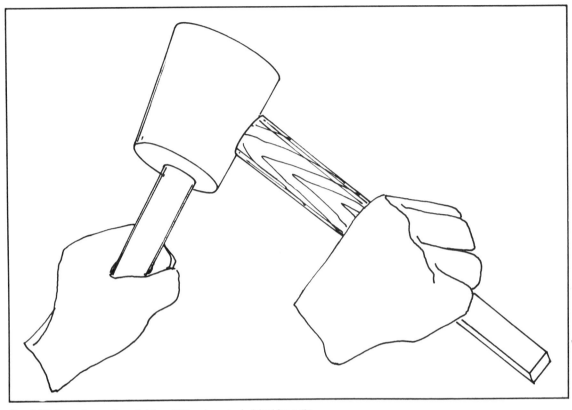

Fig. 3-37. Use of wood mallet for striking head of chisel handle.

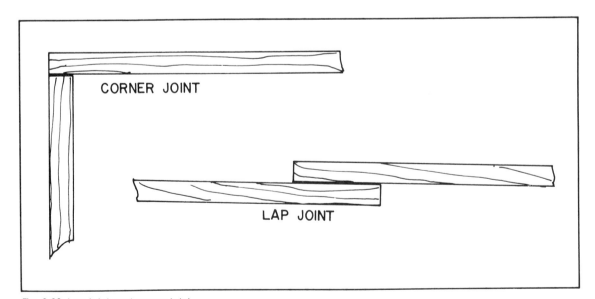

CORNER JOINT

LAP JOINT

Fig. 3-38. Lap joint and corner joint.

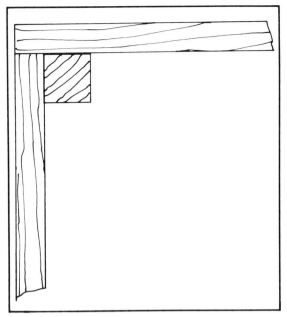

Fig. 3-39. Corner joint with post.

in Fig. 3-40. Still other possibilities include *splined joints* and *doweled joints,* but these methods are seldom used for making exercise equipment.

A common way to fasten wood is with nails; this method gives adequate strength for some exercise equipment constructions, such as attaching plywood tops to exercise steps and benches.

Another method is to use screws or lag bolts. These generally give greater holding power than nails. In most cases, pilot holes are first drilled for the screws or lag bolts. Special pilot-hole bits are available for screw fasteners.

A typical fastening is installed as follows:

- Clamp or otherwise hold the two boards in position.
- Mark the location for the screw with an awl and make the center hole in the wood to start the drilling of the pilot hole.
- Drill the pilot hole and, if you prefer, countersink and counterbore. The pilot bit used must be the correct size for the screw size and length used.
- Using a screwdriver that fits the screw, drive the screw. Hold the screwdriver firmly so that it will not slip out of the slot. In many cases, glue is applied to the contact area of the two boards before the screws are installed and tightened down.

Bolts are frequently used to attach wood parts together. Commonly used types include the flat-head machine screw, the machine bolt, the round-head bolt, the oval-head bolt, and the carriage bolt. Regular nuts can be used with washers and lock washers, or a lock nut can be used with regular washers.

Whether to use a screw or bolt depends on the particular job; bolts are generally best when considerable stresses will be involved. In most cases, tight pilot holes are drilled for bolts that

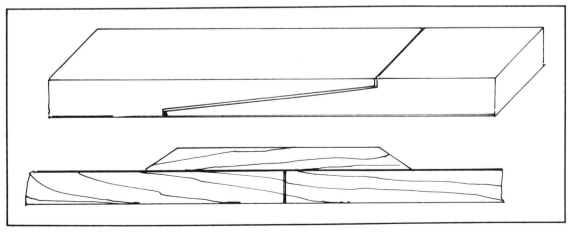

Fig. 3-40. Scarf joint and butt joint with backing board.

are not intended to be taken apart. Sometimes a loose hole is drilled when the parts are to be taken apart frequently. For permanent fastening, bolts are often used in combination with gluing.

A variety of modern glues is available for gluing wood pieces together. I have had excellent results with epoxy glues. Gluing can be with or without mechanical fasteners.

Follow the manufacturer's directions when using a particular glue. In most cases, the glue is applied to one or both contact surfaces of the wood joint and the parts are clamped together until the glue sets. For many glues, this pressure contact is necessary for a strong joint. Some glues will bond without this pressure contact, but it is generally best to clamp the joints together until the glue sets. When mechanical fasteners are also used, the mechanical fasteners will often serve to clamp the joint together under pressure until the glue sets.

Sanding and Painting

Sanding is an important operation in preparing wood for painting or varnishing. Sanding smooths the surface of wood with an abrasive material that is attached to paper and often called sandpaper. As a general rule, sanding follows the final cutting and shaping with saws, rasps, files, chisels, gouges, surfacing tools, planes, and other similar woodworking tools.

Sandpaper or abrasive paper is a strong paper that has the abrasive material glued to it. Common abrasives include flint, a soft sandstone; garnet, a hard, reddish-brown mineral; and aluminum oxide, a man-made abrasive material. Sandpaper with flint, garnet, or aluminum oxide is suitable for hand-sanding; garnet or aluminum oxide is suitable for use with power sanders.

Sandpaper, regardless of the abrasive material used, is available in various grades— coarse, medium, fine, and very fine. As a general rule, flint abrasive paper is the cheapest, but it does not last long. Garnet and aluminum oxide are usually more expensive, but last longer.

Sandpaper can be held by hand or on a sanding block. The choice really depends on what type of sanding is being done. To maintain a flat surface, a sanding block is helpful. Sanding by hand without the use of a sanding block sometimes results in a wavy surface, but this may not be critical for some sanding jobs used in making exercise equipment.

Sandpaper sometimes comes in large sheets. These can be cut or torn into smaller pieces to use for hand sanding. One way to do this is to first fold the paper with the sanded side inward in the area where you want to cut the paper. Make a sharp crease in the paper. Then unfold the paper and place the crease line at the edge of a bench. Tear the paper with a quick jerking action. As a general rule, avoid using scissors or tinsnips to cut sandpaper, as the abrasive material on the paper will quickly dull these cutting tools.

Here are some general suggestions for sanding:

- Cutting with saws, rasps, chisels, and other similar cutting tools should be finished before sanding is started. Small particles of abrasive sandpaper material are left on the wood surface when sanding is done, and these can dull cutting tools if additional cutting and shaping is done after sanding.
- Most sanding works best when done with the grain of the wood. When sanding end grain, the sanding is usually best done in one direction only.
- Use just enough pressure to make the sandpaper cut. Excessive pressure can cause scratching.
- Sanding is often best done with the wood component clamped in a vise. In some cases, the wood can be held with one hand while the sanding is done with the other hand.
- Begin with coarse sandpaper and work up gradually to finer grades. Begin with the finest grade that is practical for the particular sanding job. Coarse grades leave deep scratches, which must be removed later by finer grades of paper. Begin with the finest grade practical to keep scratches to a minimum.
- As a general rule, sanding is done to finish the surface of the wood, not to shape it. There are situations where the use of

sandpaper is the safest, however. Although usually slow, you can use it to fine shape a piece of wood.

☐ A leather or foam rubber pad can sometimes be used to advantage between a sanding block and the paper side of the sandpaper.

☐ Long sanding strokes with the grain of the wood are generally most satisfactory, although this varies, depending on the particular sanding task.

A variety of wood fillers is available for filling holes and cracks. You can also make your own filler putty by mixing sanding dust with glue. Powdered glues can be used or, perhaps better yet, epoxy glue. Epoxy generally has good bonding qualities and low shrinkage, making it ideal for filling cracks and holes in wood.

Use a wood filler or putty that is compatible with the finish that is to be applied. Some wood fillers, for example, will not take stains or will change colors when a clear finish is applied.

Wood fillers in paste form can be applied with a putty knife. Wood fillers in liquid form can often be applied with a brush. These are sometimes used for filling the pores in the surface of wood.

Always follow the manufacturer's directions for the particular product used. After the filler is dry or has set or hardened, additional sanding may be required.

Paint and varnish should be selected carefully for the particular job. *Alkyds, vinyls, polyurethanes,* and *epoxies* are four synthetic resins used in the manufacture of many modern finishes.

Select a finish that is safe to use under the conditions and with the equipment you have at hand. Read the labels on the containers to learn if there are any hazards associated with using a particular product. Follow all safety precautions for using the particular product. Take seriously any warnings that breathing vapors and fumes can be harmful to your health—if the instructions say to use adequate ventilation, do just that.

Finishes in spray cans often present special safety hazards. In some cases, the only safe way to use these is to avoid breathing the fumes and vapors entirely. This may require the use of an approved safety respirator or other special protective equipment.

Many finishes can be applied with a brush. A variety of brushes is suitable. As a general rule, quality brushes cost more than economy brushes, but they generally last longer and have superior working qualities.

For some finishes, such as epoxy, it may be more economical to purchase inexpensive throw-away brushes than to purchase the solvent for cleaning them. This is especially true of some finishes that require a catalyst or hardening agent. For most types of finishes, though, it makes sense to purchase better brushes and to clean them after use.

The cleaning solvent to use depends on the type of finish that is applied with the brush. Solvents include water, turpentine or paint thinner, alcohol, and acetone. The solvent may or may not be the same chemical that is required for thinning the finish.

By drilling a small hole through the lower portion of the handle of the brush, the brush can be suspended on a piece of wire in a can of solvent, as shown in Fig. 3-41.

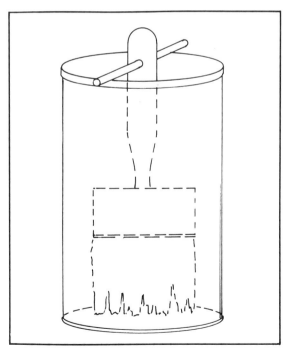

Fig. 3-41. Paint brush suspended in solvent by wire.

After a brush has been thoroughly washed in a solvent, it should then be washed in water with a detergent added. Dry the brush thoroughly. Brushes can be wrapped in wax paper for storage.

Follow the manufacturer's directions for the application of a particular finishing product. Here are some general tips and suggestions:

—Waxes, polishes, stains, and oils can often be best applied with a clean cloth rather than a brush, although some are also suitable for brush application.

—Application of various varnish, plastic, and paint finishes varies greatly. Follow the manufacturer's directions for the application of the particular product used. Some finishes require an undercoat; others don't. Some finishes require more than one coat. Usually, the first coat is allowed to dry. This is followed by light sanding, and a second coat is applied. After applying a finish, use appropriate solvent to clean the brush.

—Clear plastic finishes work well on wood surfaces of exercise equipment that is used indoors. Exterior paint or other finishes should be used for outdoor equipment. Posts and other wood components set in the ground should be treated with a wood preservative.

WORKING WITH METAL

A variety of metals can be used in the construction of exercise equipment. Most work involves cutting and shaping the metal parts and, for some constructions, brazing or welding the parts together. Almost anyone who is reasonably handy with tools can do the cutting and shaping required for the construction of the exercise equipment detailed in this book. Brazing and welding requires both special skills and equipment. If you already have brazing and welding skills and equipment, you will probably want to do this work yourself. If not, you can have this work done at a commercial shop. You can do the cutting and shaping so that only the brazing and welding needs to be done at the commercial shop to keep the cost to a minimum.

Metals

Metals are characterized by physical properties such as *hardness, color*, and *malleability*. There are two general classes of metals: *ferrous* and *nonferrous*. Ferrous metals contain iron. Nonferrous metals do not contain iron. In most cases, ferrous metals are used for constructing exercise equipment.

Cast iron is a hard, ferrous, brittle metal that contains 3 to 4 percent carbon. Cast iron is difficult to work with and heavy, limiting it's usefulness in constructing home exercise equipment.

Wrought iron has most of the carbon removed. It is tough, yet bends easily with or without heat. It is also easy to weld. Wrought iron can be used for making frames and support arms on exercise equipment parts that have light or moderate stresses placed on them.

Steel is a mixture of iron and an alloy, either carbon and/or some other element or elements. The alloying elements are used to add desired characteristics to iron for particular applications. Carbon steel is iron with carbon as the alloying element. Mild steels are low carbon steels that contain less than 0.30 percent carbon. Low carbon steel is available in sheet and band iron and in many sizes and shapes of rods, bars, and pipes. Mild steel coated with zinc is often called *galvanized iron*.

Also useful for constructing exercise equipment are medium carbon (0.30 to 0.60 percent carbon), and high carbon (0.60 to 1.50 percent carbon) steel.

Other alloys, such as manganese, chromium, nickel, molybdenum, vanadium, and tungsten, make the steel harder, tougher, and stronger. These steels are generally more expensive and difficult to work than are carbon steels, which limits their usefulness for making home exercise equipment.

Cutting

When constructing exercise equipment, it will often be necessary to cut metal bar stock, rod, pipe, angle iron, and other shapes. Hacksaws can be used for cutting these bench metals. A hacksaw has a handle, a frame and a blade, as

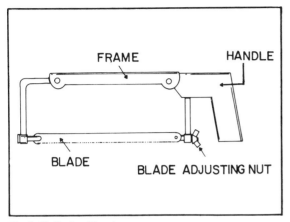

Fig. 3-42. Parts of hacksaw.

shown in Fig. 3-42. The blades are measured by points per inch. The number of teeth per inch is one less than the number of points, as shown in Fig. 3-43. The 11-point blade shown has 10 teeth per inch. Different numbers of points are used for different metals. For example, 24 teeth per inch (25-point blade) is suitable for cutting angle iron and other easy-to-cut metals; 18 teeth per inch (19-point blade) is suitable for cutting high carbon steel; and 14 teeth per inch (15-point blade) is suitable for cutting mild steel.

Safety is an important consideration when using a hacksaw, mainly because of the possibility of a blade breaking, which could cause an injury. To avoid breaking blades, adjust the blade properly in the hacksaw frame. Adjust tension on the blade until it is tight in the frame, but not so tight that breakage will occur around the ends of the blade. The teeth should point away from the handle. Once the blade is in the frame, the wingnut by the handle is used to tighten the blade. The blade should be straight

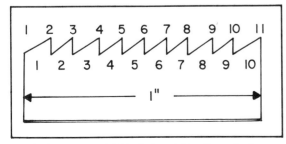

Fig. 3-43. Eleven-point blade has 10 teeth per inch.

from one end to the other in the saw frame, but can be turned at any desired angle.

Select a blade that is designed for the particular job you intend to do. The blade should be sharp and in good condition. Hacksaw blades are usually not resharpened; damaged and worn blades are usually discarded and replaced with new ones.

When sawing, apply only light pressure and do not twist the saw. Do not saw too rapidly. If the blade becomes loose in the frame, stop sawing and readjust the blade. If the metal slips, twisting can cause the blade to break.

The metal to be cut should be fastened in a vise or otherwise securely held in position for sawing so that vibrations will be kept to a minimum. When using a vise, for example, have the line you will be sawing along just outside the vise jaws.

Stand a comfortable distance in front of the work and hold the hacksaw in both hands, as shown in Fig. 3-44. Keep one hand on the handle and the other hand on the far end of the hacksaw frame. Start the cut on the backstroke, applying only light pressure. After the saw cut has been started, apply pressure only on forward strokes of the blade. Pressure should be sufficient to keep the blade cutting throughout the forward stroke of the saw. Both too much and too little pressure can cause the blade to wear more rapidly than normal. The pressure is released on the backstroke.

Special tungsten-carbide hacksaw blades are available for sawing hard materials such as stainless steel. Unlike ordinary hacksaw blades, these special blades cut on both the forward and back strokes. These blades, while more expensive than ordinary hacksaw blades, can be worth the cost when sawing hard metals.

Metal-cutting chisels can be used to cut or shear metal. These chisels are often called *cold chisels*. A flat chisel (Fig. 2-36) is useful for general cutting. As a rule, a cold chisel can be used to cut any metal that is softer than the material from which the chisel is made.

To shear or cut metal, select a flat cold chisel that is large enough for the particular job. You will also need a hammer that matches the chisel. Larger chisels require heavier hammers. The piece of metal to be cut should be clamped in a

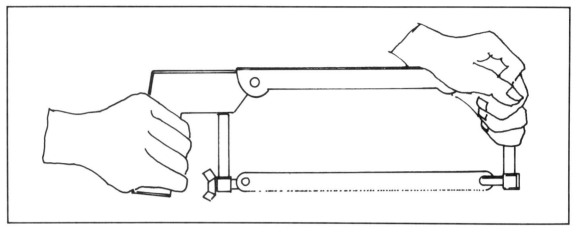

Fig. 3-44. Basic hacksaw grip.

metal vise so that the cutting line is just above the jaws of the vise, as shown in Fig. 3-45. Wear protective eye goggles when using a cold chisel. The chisel is usually held in the left hand with thumb and first finger about an inch from the striking head of the chisel. Hold the chisel steady, but not too tightly. Relax your fingers to the point where, if the hammer accidently strikes the fingers, the fingers will slide down the chisel. Watch the cutting edge of the chisel when striking the head of the chisel with the hammer.

The chisel is held on top of the jaw of the vise. Hold the hammer in your right hand and strike the head of the chisel. Move the chisel

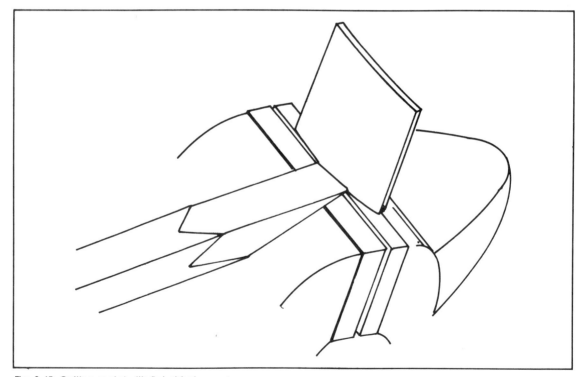

Fig. 3-45. Cutting metal with flat chisel.

along the metal cutting line and repeat hammer strikes at each position, overlapping the chisel blade with the previous cut.

Cold chisels can also be used to cut round stock. Mark the round stock where the cut is desired. Place the round stock on top of an anvil or other solid metal surface. Place the cutting edge of the chisel on the mark, hold the chisel in a vertical position, and strike the chisel with the hammer, using a series of blows. When the round stock is nearly cut into two pieces, use easy hammer strikes to avoid damage to the anvil or other solid metal surface that you are using. In some cases, especially with heavy round stock, the cut can be made half way through; then turn the material over and finish the cut from the opposite side.

A mushroomed head on a cold chisel can be dangerous, as pieces of metal may fly off as the chisel head is struck with a hammer. Regrind the chisel head to the original shape.

When straight cuts are made on pipe, a pipe cutter can be used. These generally have cutting wheels mounted in an adjustable clamping arrangement. The cutting wheels are clamped around the pipe and the device is rotated. The clamp is gradually tightened until the pipe is cut in two.

Using Files

Metal cutting files are available in a variety of cuts, shapes, and sizes. The three basic cuts are single, double, and curved tooth (Fig. 3-46). Metal files are available in a variety of shapes, including flat, square, triangular, half-round, and round. Select a file that is designed for the particular job at hand. A file should have a handle.

For proper filing, the teeth of the file should be kept clean. A special wire brush called a *file card* can be used to remove clogging materials from the file teeth.

The metal to be cut should be clamped in a vise or otherwise secured. Straight or cross filing is done with forward strokes, often the length of the cutting blade, and with the file held at a slight angle to the metal being filed. Grip the file handle in your right hand and apply pressure to the end of the file with your left hand, as shown in Fig. 3-47. The left hand is also used to guide

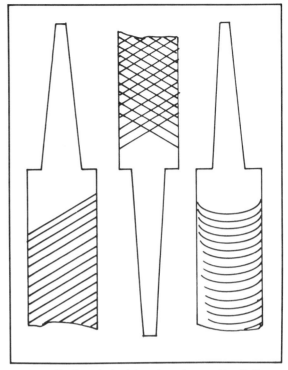

Fig. 3-46. Single-cut, double-cut, and curved-tooth files.

the file. Pressure is applied on the forward strokes to do the cutting and then released on the return strokes. On hard metals, the file can be lifted from the metal on the return strokes.

Apply just enough pressure to keep the file cutting efficiently. To file a flat, square surface, avoid letting the file seesaw or rock. It takes considerable practice to keep the surface true.

Draw filing is another method for filing. The file is held sideways and alternately pushed forward and then drawn back across the metal, as shown in Fig. 3-47. A single-cut file is usually used. Using this method, it is fairly easy to hold the file steady, making a smooth surface possible. Draw filing does tend to produce sharp edges, however, which can be removed by holding the file at an angle and lightly draw filing the edges.

Using Power Grinders

Bench-mounted power grinders are extremely useful tools when grinding metal for exercise equipment constructions. While it is possible to

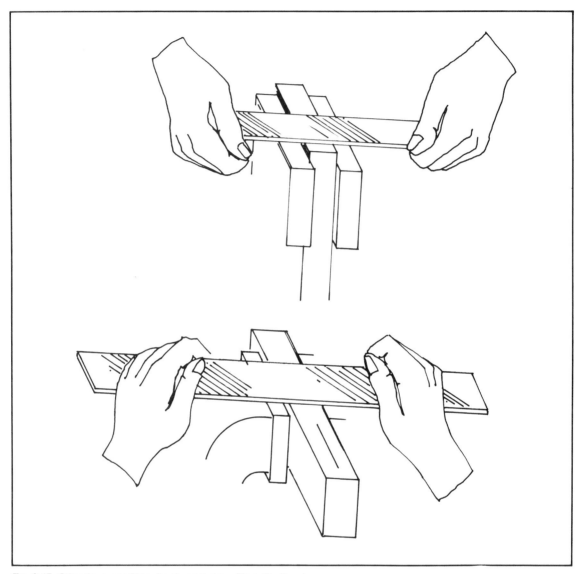

Fig. 3-47. Grips for cross filing (top), and draw filing (bottom).

do the same jobs with files, the power grinders usually make the work much faster and easier.

Safety is extremely important when using power grinders. Check grinding wheels before installing them on the grinder. Follow the instructions of the manufacturer for using the particular tool. Wear proper clothing: there should be no loose sleeves or other clothing that could get caught in the grinder motor or wheels. Do not wear rings or other jewelry while using power grinders. A wheel guard, tool rest, and safety shield should be in place and properly adjusted. For many grinding jobs, the tool rest is adjusted to within ⅛-inch of the face of the grinding wheel and set level with the center of the grinding wheel. Wear safety goggles. Stand to one side when starting the motor in case the grinding wheel is defective and flies apart. This is rare, but it has happened.

Here are some tips for grinding:

- Grinding is generally done only on the outer face of the wheel. Do not use the side of the wheel unless the grinder and grinding wheel are designed and set up for this.
- Keep the metal being ground at low temperature by using water or other coolant.
- Adjust the tool rest so that the metal to be ground is at the centerline of the wheel.
- To grind a straight edge on metal stock, place the metal on the tool rest. Keep the edge that is being worked parallel to the centerline of the grinding wheel, and work the metal stock back and forth across the grinding wheel.

Another job that is often done is to grind a bevel edge. Rest the metal stock on the tool rest and angle the end to be ground upward against the grinding wheel. Maintain the angle for the desired bevel and work the metal stock back and forth across the grinding wheel.

A rounded edge can also be ground on metal. The metal is positioned on the grinding wheel in the same manner as for grinding a straight edge, but this time the metal is swung back and forth in an arc.

The grinding wheel is useful not only for shaping metal parts, but also for sharpening a number of tools, such as wood chisels, plane blades, and drill bits. Special guides are available for holding twist drill bits at desired angles to sharpen them on grinding wheels. Many sharpening jobs are started on grinding wheels and then finished by hand on sharpening or oil stones.

Drilling

While a limited amount of metal drilling can be done with hand drills, this isn't very practical. While it is usually fairly easy to drill a hole in a soft metal like aluminum with a hand drill, this can be a real challenge with stainless steel and other hard metals. The low cost and easy availability of electric drills makes them very practical for constructing home exercise equipment.

There are two basic types of electric drills: the hand drill and the drill press. Both types work in the same basic way, except that the hand drill is held and guided by hand while the drill press is mounted on a mechanical guide. The drill press allows more accurate drilling, but is also more expensive to buy. There are also drill press stands that use standard electric hand drills.

The general steps in drilling a hole through a piece of metal are as follows:

- Mark the desired location for the hole with a center punch. This will form a seat for the drill point and prevent the drill point from "walking off" the mark.
- The metal is usually secured by some mechanical means such as in a vise or with clamps. Make certain that the metal is secure. Metal coming loose while drilling can result in accidents.
- Select the correct drill size. Gauges are available for measuring drill sizes.
- Install the drill in the chuck of the drill. The drill should always be unplugged when this is being done. Use a chuck key to secure the drill in the chuck.
- Wear safe working clothes. Loose sleeves could get caught in the drill. Wear eye protection.
- Plug the drill in and position the point of the drill on the center punch mark.
- Start the drill motor and apply pressure on the drill.
- While aluminum, brass, and other soft metals can usually be drilled without the use of a cutting oil to cool the drill bit while drilling, most hard metals require a cutting oil for proper drilling—even for aluminum and brass a cutting oil can be helpful. Kerosene is often used as a cutting oil.

It is extremely important to select twist drill bits that can take considerable heat without becoming dull or weakening them. High speed twist drills made from an alloy containing tungsten, chromium, and vanadium work well.

Special problems are encountered when drilling stainless steel and other hard metals. Low cutting speeds are generally used, and this requires either a low speed or variable speed electric drill. If possible, use a drill press stand for holding the portable drill, or better yet, use a shop drill press.

Bending Metal

In many cases, metal can be cold bent by clamping the metal in a vise and bending it by hand or with hammer force, as shown in Fig. 3-48. Metal can also be bent by first heating it with a torch or by other means. In both cases, care must be taken not to weaken the metal beyond allowable limits for the particular use.

Assembly of Metal Components

Metal components used for making exercise equipment can be assembled in a variety of ways, including the use of rivets, bolts and other

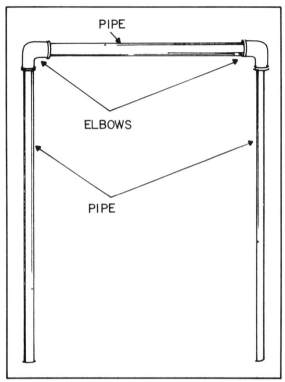

Fig. 3-49. Pipe and pipe fittings with threaded joints.

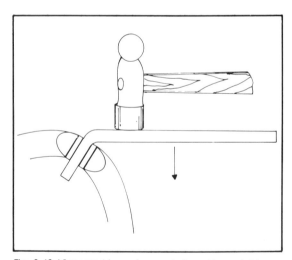

Fig. 3-48. Vise used to make angle bend in metal bar.

mechanical fasteners, pipe fittings, brazing, and welding. If pipe fittings are used, the parts are then threaded together, as shown in Fig. 3-49. The joints can be reinforced by brazing or welding. Another method of joining pipe sections is by brazing or welding. For a corner joint, the pipe ends can be cut at 45 degree angles. The cutting can be done with a hacksaw, as detailed above, or with a cutting torch. You can either do the brazing or welding yourself, or you can have it done for you at a commercial shop.

Chapter 4

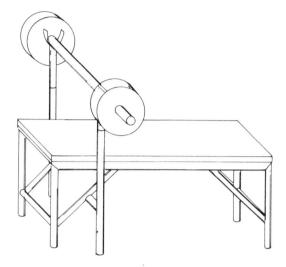

Basic Exercise Equipment

PLANS AND INSTRUCTIONS FOR MAKING A VARIETY of basic exercise equipment are given in this chapter. All of the equipment described is free-standing in the sense that no floor, wall, or ceiling attachments are required, nothing is set down in the ground. Many of the items are portable; however, these can still be important parts of permanent home exercise gyms. Some of the items, such as weight training benches, form the basis of some of the more complicated equipment covered in later chapters.

JUMP ROPES

Jump ropes provide endurance exercise that you can do in a limited space. While complete books have been written about entire exercise programs based on jumping rope, I believe that this form of exercise, for variety if nothing else, is best combined with other exercises to form a complete workout program. While a simple piece of rope can be used, the jumping rope shown in Fig. 4-1, with swivel handles and tubing used to weight the center section of the rope, makes rope jumping smoother, easier, and

a lot more fun. Manufactured jump ropes of good quality are available for about $5 and up, so you won't want to go to too much trouble and expense to make one. If you purchase a jump rope, make certain that you get one that has the swivel feature and is both long enough and heavy enough for easy jumping. Most jumping ropes made for small children will not suffice for adults, as these are usually both too short and too light in weight.

To make your own, the wooden handles are best turned on a wood lathe. If you don't have the equipment and/or the know-how for doing this, there are a number of alternative possibilities. You can shape them from wood dowels with wood rasps, files, surfacing tools, or other suitable shaping tools; or you can use the handles from rolling pins or other items of approximately the desired shape or that can be modified to the right shape. In a typical secondhand store, you will probably see a number of items that have possibilities. Still another possibility is to use wood dowels with bicycle handlebar grips placed over them for jump rope handles.

Large wood screws with round heads are

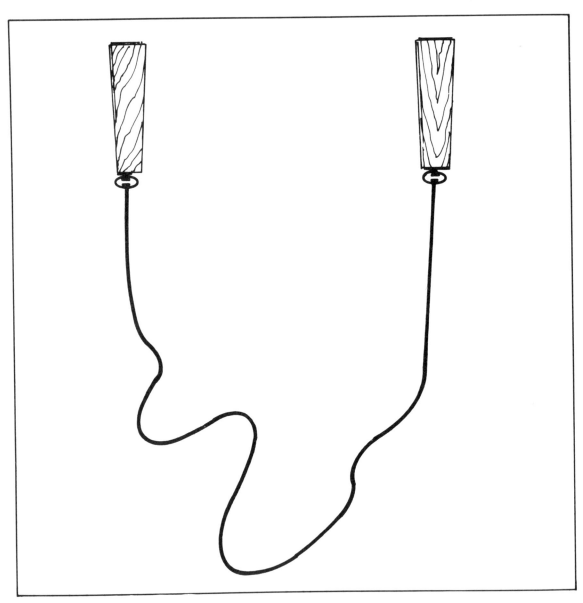

Fig. 4-1. Jump rope with swivel handles.

threaded into pilot holes in the handles to attach the wire swivel pieces. The swivel pieces are shaped from stiff wire to the pattern shown in Fig. 4-2.

While various sizes and kinds of rope can be used, I have found that ½-inch diameter cotton, polyester, or nylon works well. If the rope is too light for easy jumping, a section of soft flexible plastic tubing that will just fit over the rope can be used to give added weight in the center, as shown. The rope length should be such that when you stand and hold the ends of the rope in your hands at chest level, the hanging center section will just reach the floor.

Large washers are first placed on the mounting screws. The screws are then passed

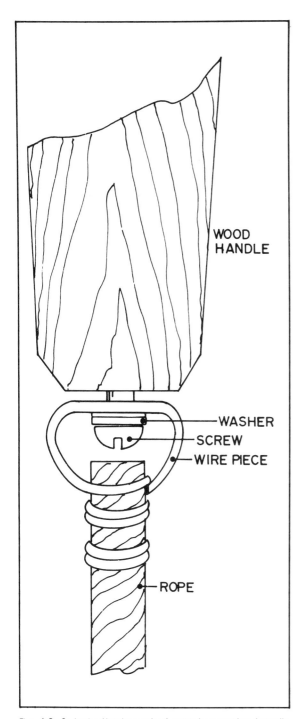

Fig. 4-2. Swivel attachment of rope to wooden handle showing wood screw threaded into pilot hole and swivel piece shaped from stiff wire.

through the mounting loops in the swivel wires and threaded into the pilot holes in the handles (Fig. 4-2). These should be tightened only to the point where the swivels will still turn freely. The rope ends are then crimped to the wire swivels, as shown. Make the crimps light and try the jumping rope out to make certain that you have the desired length of rope. Make adjustments as necessary. When everything seems right, crimp the rope tightly in the wire pieces. This completes the construction of a basic jump rope.

ELASTIC OR SPRING CHEST PULL

Chest pull devices with elastic cords (Fig. 4-3) or springs are popular strength exercise devices. Basically, the device consists of two handles arranged so that one or more elastic cords or springs can be connected between the handles. The device can be used not only in front of the body, but also overhead and behind the back, making possible strength exercises for a variety of muscle groups. I recommend that you use elastic cords rather than springs, as it is possible to pinch your skin in the springs. Springs are found on a number of manufactured models, however, so I assume that they can be used with reasonable safety.

The construction details for making a chest pull exerciser handle are shown in Fig. 4-4. The handle rods are shaped from 3/16-inch diameter mild steel rod. The loops (usually five or six) for attaching the elastic cords or springs can be bent around a steel rod. The handles themselves are made from sections of 1/4-inch inside diameter pipe with a thick-walled rubber or plastic hose placed over it. An alternative is to use 1-inch diameter hardwood dowels with a hole drilled through the centers.

Regardless of the handles used, insert the ends of the shaped handle rods in the end holes and bend the rods together so that the handles will stay in place.

Elastic cords can be purchased with hooks already attached to the ends. These are ideal for use on the chest pull exerciser. An alternative is to use screen door springs. If the springs are used, small "S" hooks can be used to make the connections to the handle loops, as shown in Fig. 4-4. These arrangements allow easy addition and removal of the elastic cords or springs

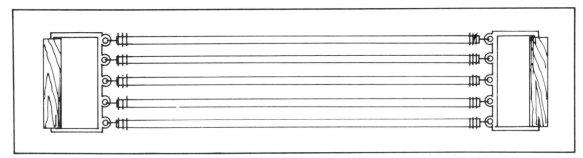

Fig. 4-3. Chest pull device with elastic cords.

so that various numbers can be used, depending on the desired resistance for a particular exercise. This completes the construction of a basic chest pull exerciser.

ISOMETRIC ROPE AND CHAIN PULL DEVICES

Isometric exercise, which is essentially pulling or pushing against an immovable object, may have some exercise value, although it has not lived up to the ideal strength building exercise made in early claims. The isometric rope device and isometric chain device (Fig. 4-5), which are essentially the same except for the rope or chain, can be used for a variety of isometric exercises. For example, by adjusting the length of the rope or chain for various angles of elbow bends, a variety of isometric curling exercises can be done, such as shown in Fig. 4-6.

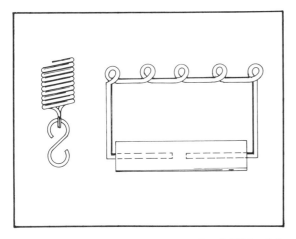

Fig. 4-4. Chest pull exerciser handle. Small "S" hook is used to connect spring to loop in handle.

For both a rope and chain exerciser, a $2 \times 6 \times 18$ = inch long piece of hardwood can be used. For a rope attachment, a $5/16$-inch U-bolt that is 4 inches long is installed in the center of the board, as shown in Fig. 4-7. Holes are drilled for the U-bolt to pass through the wood. Larger holes are drilled on one side to a depth equal to the width of the nut and backing washing so that the end of the U-bolts will not extend all the way through the wood when installed, as shown. A welded chain link that will just fit over the U-bolt is used for attaching the rope and making easy adjustments when the rope is slack (Fig. 4-8). The rope used on the device shown is $3/8$-inch diameter polyester rope, but nylon can also be used. The rope should be about $7\frac{1}{2}$ feet long. The handle is made a piece of 1-inch outside diameter pipe that is 18 inches long (Fig. 4-9). Drill a $3/8$-inch hole in the center of one side of the pipe. Thread the rope through the hole and through and out one end of the pipe. Make a stop-knot in the end of the rope, then pull the rope back out of the hole until the stop knot is inside the pipe over the hole. If desired, non-skid pads can be cemented to the upper side of the wooden foot base.

The chain pull exerciser uses the same base, except that a $5/16$-inch diameter eye bolt with an open, non-welded ring is used in the base instead of the U-bolt, as shown in Fig. 4-10. The eye is opened slightly to allow you to slip chain links over it.

A chain with 2-inch welded links that is about $7\frac{1}{2}$ feet long is used. The handle is a piece of 1-inch outside diameter steel pipe that is 18 inches long. A $5/16$-inch hole is drilled through both walls of the center of the pipe for attachment of a $5/16$-inch diameter eye bolt, as shown in

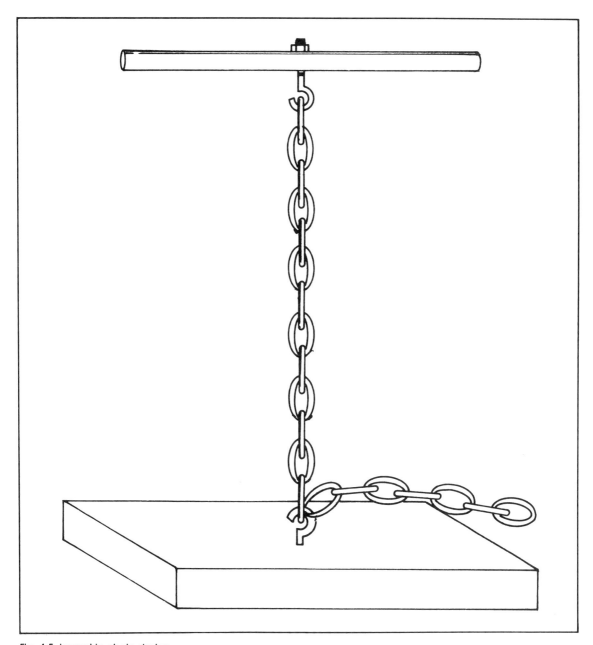

Fig. 4-5. Isometric chain device.

Fig. 4-11. A backing washer and lock washer should be used under the nut. Tighten the nut down, then cut off excess threads, and file smooth. The eye bolt should be opened slightly to allow slipping in chain links.

The length of the chain used between the foot base and the hand bar can be adjusted by changing the chain link connections at either the foot base eye bolt or the hand bar eye bolt. This allows quick adjustments with slack in the

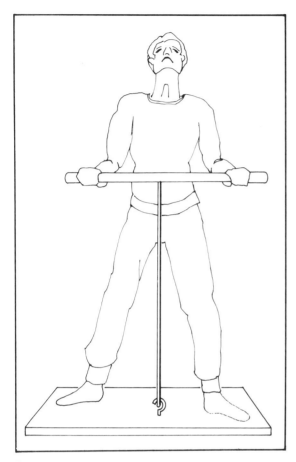

Fig. 4-6. Use of isometric device for curling exercise.

chain, yet gives a good attachment when tension is placed on the device for isometric exercise. As with the rope arrangement, you may want to cement non-skid pads to the upper side of the wooden base to give better footing.

DUMBBELLS AND BARBELLS

Consider practicality before constructing your own dumbbells and/or barbells. Some manufactured dumbbells and barbells are available at discount prices. Used dumbbells and barbells can be even cheaper.

Compare this with the cost of the materials and the time involved in making them to see if it is worth it in your particular case.

While the manufactured weights are usually cast iron or steel, it is usually easier to use cement to make your own. You can use a ready-mix cement, or you can add sand and gravel to cement, as desired. While a variety of mold forms can be used, I prefer to use plastic or metal cans or containers, which I leave in place after the cement has hardened.

While the weight will vary depending on the cement mix and other factors, a cylinder of cement 6 inches in diameter and 2½ inches thick will weigh about 5 pounds; 10 pounds if 5 inches thick. A cylinder of cement 10 inches in diameter and 2½ inches thick will weigh about 15 pounds; 20 pounds if 3 inches thick; and 25 pounds if 4 inches thick. Keep in mind that these figures are approximations.

To construct a 10-pound dumbbell, as shown in Fig. 4-12, you will need a 1-inch inside diameter section of pipe that is 12 inches long, two plastic or metal containers with closed bottoms and open tops, heavy wire, and wire mesh. Drill holes in near the ends of the pipe to pass the heavy wires through, as shown in Fig. 4-13. Then position the pipe in one of the cans or containers and prop or clamp it in place in the center of the container and perpendicular to it, as shown in Fig. 4-14. Place wire mesh in the container to reinforce the cement. You will not need much for these small weights, but when you construct heavier and larger ones, the wire mesh reinforcement becomes more important.

Mix the ready-mix cement or a mixture of cement, sand, and fine gravel and pour it into the container, working the cement down inside the container through the wire mesh. Fill the container to the top and scrape off excess, level with the top of the container (Fig. 4-15). Allow the cement to harden overnight or longer. Then install the weight on the other end in the same manner.

Since dumbbells are usually used in pairs, you will probably want to make two of the same size and weight at the same time.

Using this same technique, you can make dumbbells of lesser and greater weights and with shorter and longer handles, as desired. While it is also possible to make dumbbells with removable weights so that the weight can be changed (using collars tapped for thumb screws (see Fig. 4-20), this is generally more trouble than it is worth for small dumbbells. For general exercise at the

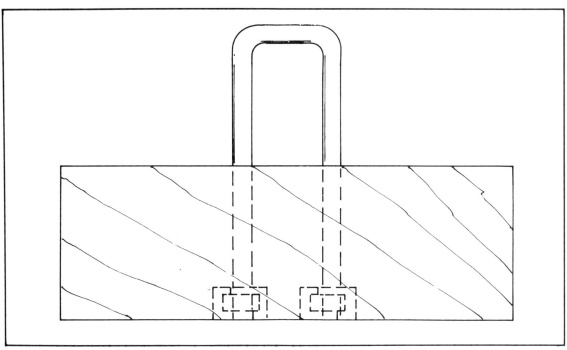

Fig. 4-7. U-bolt installed in wood base.

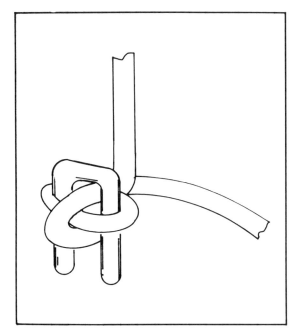

Fig. 4-8. Welded chain link is used over U-bolt to form rope locking device, and rope is locked in set position.

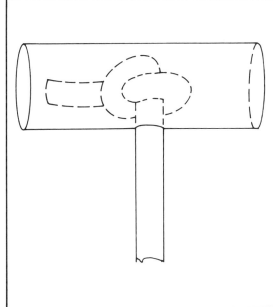

Fig. 4-9. Attachment of rope to pipe handle.

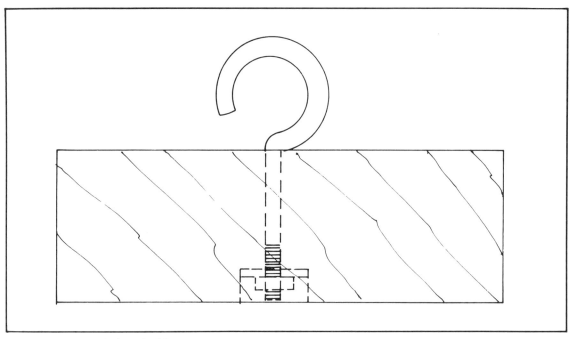

Fig. 4-10. Attachment of eye bolt to wood base.

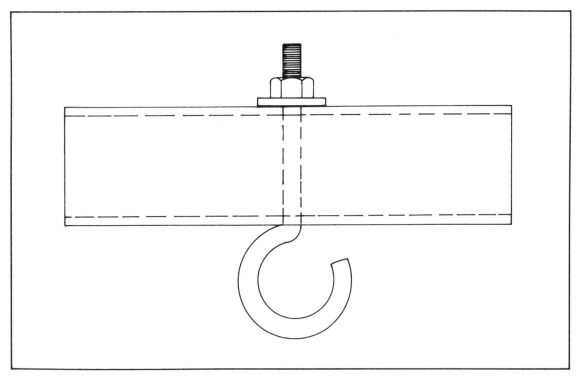

Fig. 4-11. Attachment of eye bolt to pipe handle.

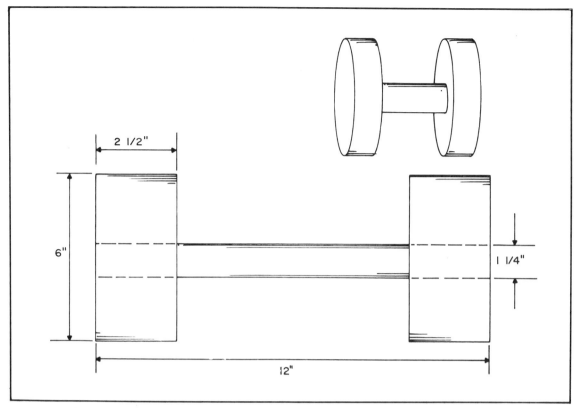

Fig. 4-12. Plan for 10-pound dumbbell.

beginning stages, pairs of 5-, 10-, 15-, and 20-pound dumbbells will probably be useful. I suggest that you avoid using heavy weights for general exercise and physical fitness training, at least in the beginning.

Barbells can be made in a similar manner, except that a longer bar (usually at least 4 feet long and often 6 feet or even more) and usually heavier weights are used. Also, you will usually only need one pair of each different weight. Figure 4-16 shows the construction of a typical barbell with a set weight. To give added strength, a steel bar rather than hollow pipe is usually used.

You can also make barbells with weight plates that can be added or subtracted from the bar to give desired weight. See Figs. 4-17 and 4-18. This allows one bar to serve for a variety of weights. The usual arrangement is to clamp the weight plates between collars at each end of the bar. The cement weights are then constructed with holes in them so that they can be slipped over the bar. One way to do this is to place a section of metal tubing that will just slip over the pipe bar in the plastic or metal container, as shown in Fig. 4-19. Position the wire mesh and make certain that the metal insert is exactly centered. The mix and pour the cement in place.

Collars can be made from sections of pipe that will just fit over the bar. A hole is drilled through one side of each separate collar, which is tapped for a thumb screw or L-bolt or, better, for brazing or welding a nut to the collar for a thumb screw or L-bolt (Fig. 4-20).

In order to use fewer collars, the inside weights can be attached to the bar, as detailed previously for a set weight barbell, except that the weights are placed a foot or more from the ends of the bar to give space for adding additional weights.

Tricycle wheels, which can often be purchased used, can also be used as forms for

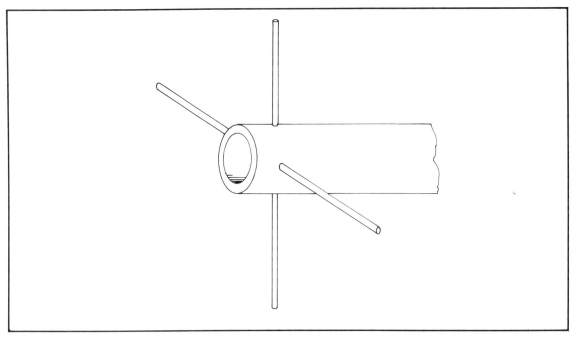

Fig. 4-13. Holes are drilled in pipe for wire reinforcements.

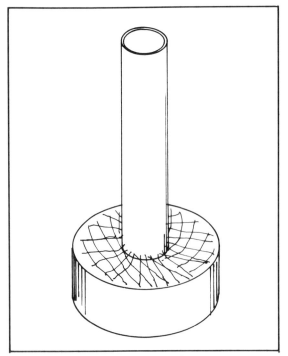

Fig. 4-14. One end of pipe is positioned in container, and wire mesh is used to reinforce cement.

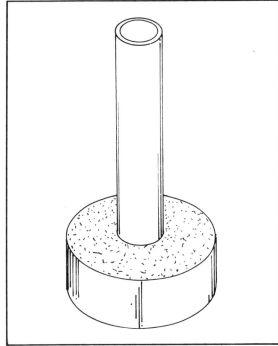

Fig. 4-15. Container is filled with cement and excess is scraped off.

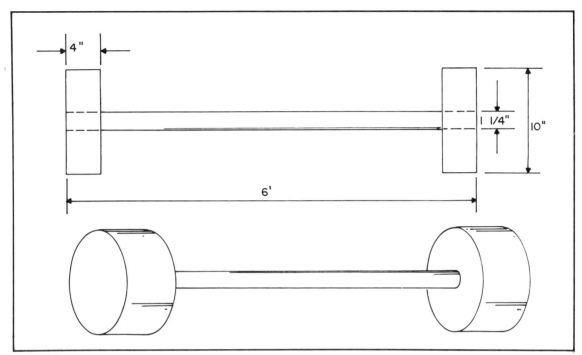

Fig. 4-16. Plan for 50-pound barbell.

making cement weights. The tires, which are left in place, give a protective cushion in case you drop the bar.

Still another idea is to use polyester resin, which must be catalyzed before use, mixed with iron boiler punchings instead of cement to form the weights. This mixture can be formed in molds similarly to cement.

BASIC WEIGHT TRAINING BENCHES

A flat bench (Fig. 4-21) is a basic piece of equipment used for weight training, (Fig. 4-22).

The bench should be a convenient size and height, sturdy, and with a padded top.

The bench legs and base can be constructed of wood or metal, the choice depending on available materials and tools.

The construction details for a wood base are shown in Fig. 4-23. All parts of the base are cut from 2 × 4-inch wood stock. Assemble with slotted round-head bolts and washers, with the nuts countersunk to just below the surface of the wood, as shown in Fig. 4-24. An alternate method is to use machine bolts with hex heads and washers and countersink both the head and

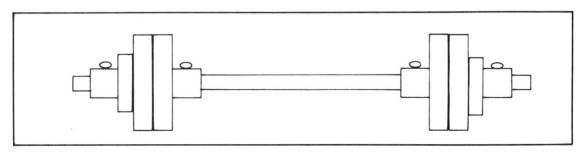

Fig. 4-17. Barbell with removable weight plates.

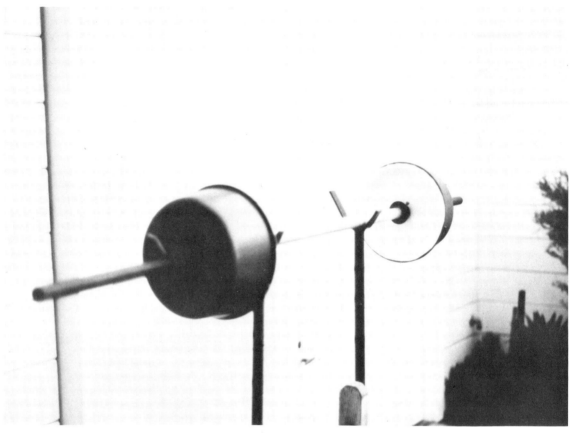

Fig. 4-18. Barbell weights constructed from plastic pans filled with cement.

nut ends below the surface of the wood, as shown in Fig. 4-25. Assembly can use lag bolts, screws, or nails, but these methods are generally less satisfactory than regular bolts. If lag bolts, screws, or nails are used, I suggest that you also

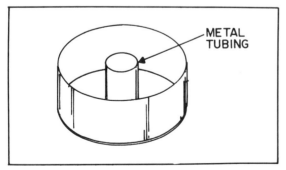

Fig. 4-19. Section of metal tubing that will just fit over metal bar is placed in container.

epoxy glue the joints. Regardless of the assembly method, it's important that you don't have any protrusions with sharp edges or corners, like bolt threads, extending beyond the surface of the wood.

The above design for the construction of a wood base is only one of many possibilities. You can use any construction design that will give adequate strength and rigidity.

After the wood base has been completed, it can be sanded and varnished or painted as desired.

The base for the bench can also be constructed from ¾-inch inside diameter steel pipe, as shown in Fig. 4-26. This construction involves brazing or welding, which you can have done at a commercial shop if you don't have the skill and/or equipment for doing this work yourself. It will usually cost much less if you

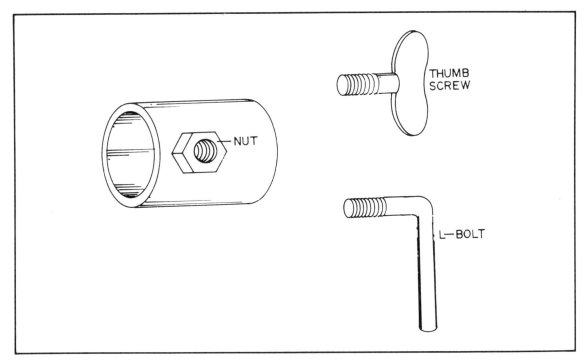

Fig. 4-20. Barbell collar.

have all the parts cut and fitted before you go to the commercial shop so that only the welding need be done.

The above design for the construction of a metal base is only one of many possibilities. You can use any construction design that will give adequate strength and rigidity.

When the brazing or welding has been completed, the joints can be ground, filed, and sanded as necessary. The base can then be

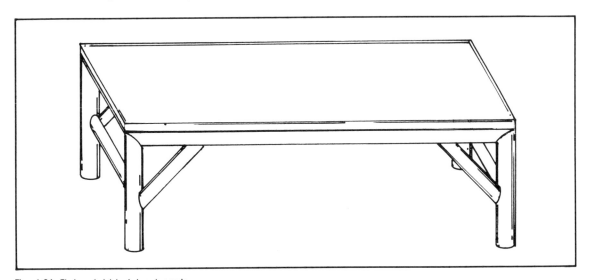

Fig. 4-21. Flat weight training bench.

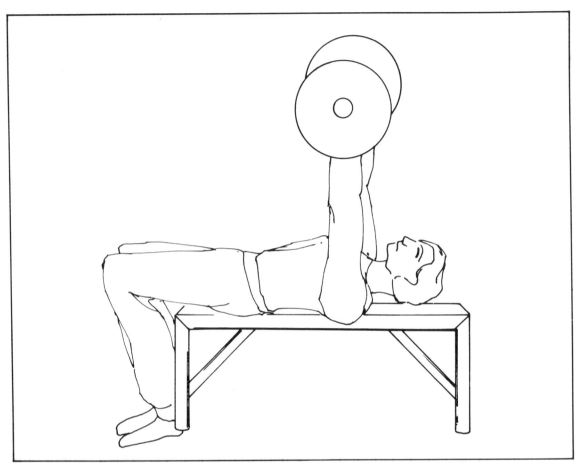

Fig. 4-22. Use of flat bench for weight exercise.

painted as desired. Rubber or plastic leg caps can be added to the legs.

For both the wood and metal bases, the bench top is made of ½-inch plywood with two 1 × 2-inch stringers attached to the bottom, as shown in Figs. 4-23 and 4-26. Cut a 1-inch or thicker section of foam rubber the same size as the wood top (14 inches by 48 inches in the plans shown) and cement this to the wood (Fig. 4-27). Cover with fabric backed vinyl or other suitable material, folding the edges around and under the wood base and attaching the material to the underside of the base around the edge with staples or tacks.

The completed bench top is attached to a wood base with screws passing through the stringers into the top side beams of the base (as shown in Fig. 4-28) and to a metal base by bolts passing through the top metal side beams of the base through holes in the stringers, as shown in Fig. 4-29.

A popular addition to a basic flat weight training bench is a barbell stand to hold the weight, as shown in Fig. 4-30. This provides a convenient means for starting bench presses. After the exercise set has been completed, the weight can be returned to the stand.

While the distance from the sides of the 14-inch wide bench to the arms for the bar stand can vary, I have found 6 inches outward on both sides, Fig. 4-31, to be about right for most applications. The stand should also be set inward from the end of the bench ample distance so that the barbell placed on the rack will not

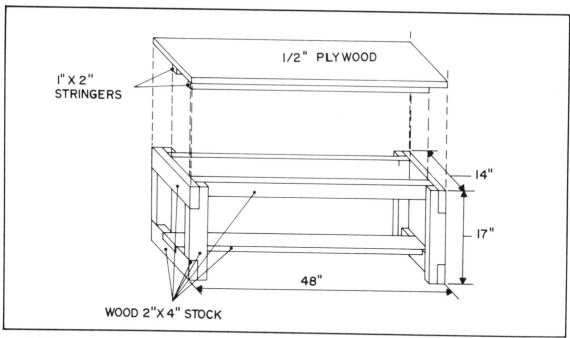

Fig. 4-23. Construction of base for flat bench from wood.

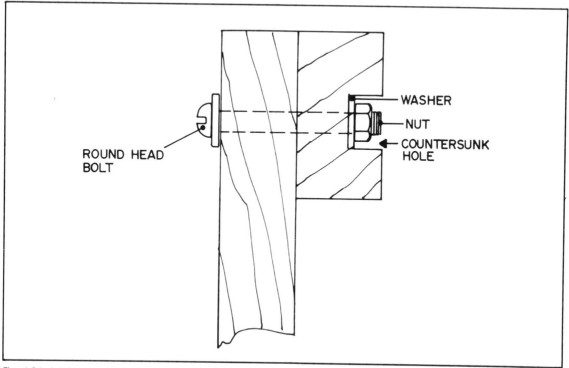

Fig. 4-24. Joining wood parts with slotted round head bolt.

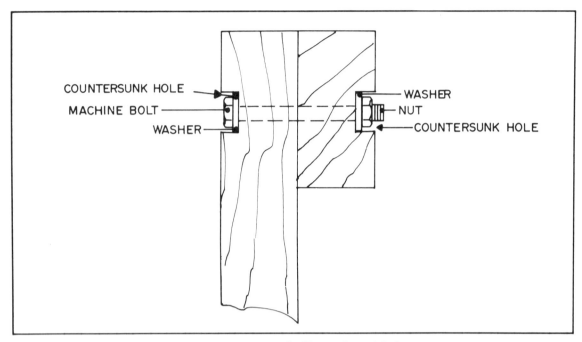

Fig. 4-25. Joining wood parts with hex head machine bolt with countersunk holes.

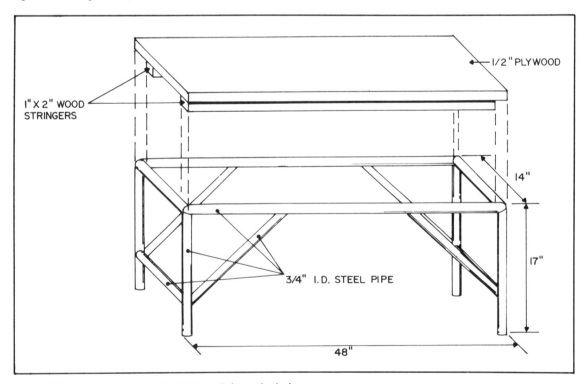

Fig. 4-26. Construction of base for flat bench from steel pipe.

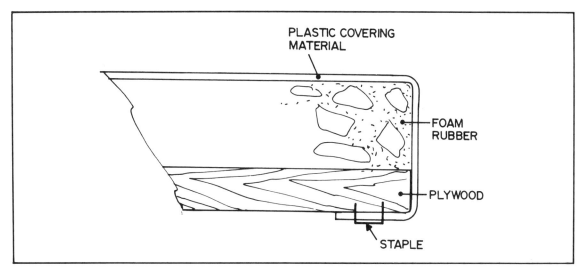

Fig. 4-27. Bench top is padded with foam rubber and covered with plastic material.

tend to tip the end of the bench. The height of the bar brackets above the bench can be at a fixed level or adjustable, as desired.

Figures 4-32 and 4-33 show the construction of wooden bar bracket arms at a fixed height for attachment to the wooden base detailed above.

Adjustable arms are shown in Fig. 4-34. For either arrangement, the lower ends of the arms form additional legs for the bench to give added support when the barbell is placed on the rack.

The bar brackets for wooden arms are bent from $2 \times \frac{1}{4}$-inch steel bar stock, as shown in Fig.

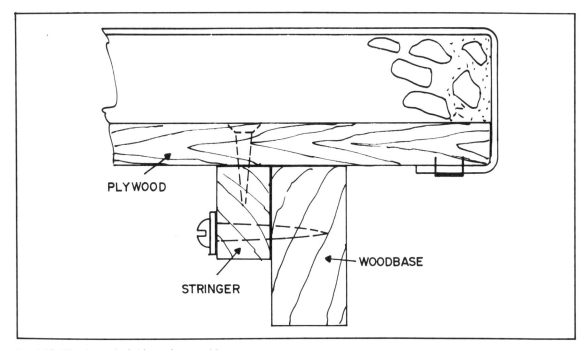

Fig. 4-28. Attachment of stringer to wood base.

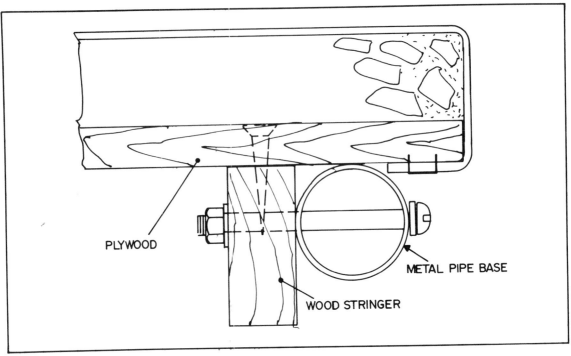

PLYWOOD

METAL PIPE BASE

WOOD STRINGER

Fig. 4-29. Attachment of stringer to metal base.

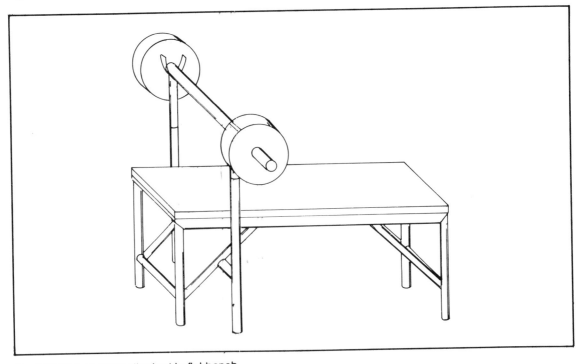

Fig. 4-30. Weight stand attached to flat bench.

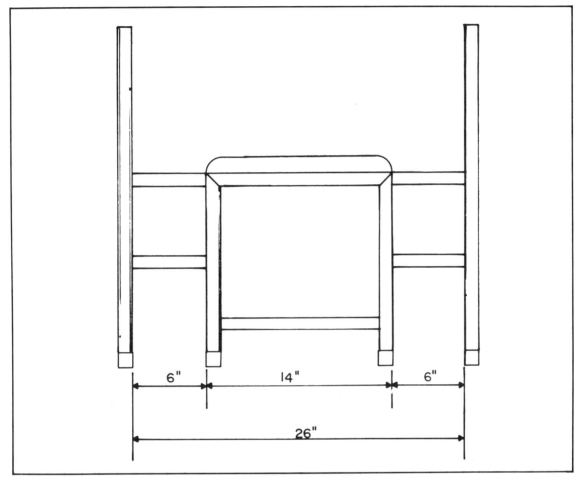

Fig. 4-31. Placement of weight stand arms 6 inches from sides of bench.

4-35. You will need two of these, one for each arm. The upper ends of the arms are cut to the curved pattern shown. The brackets are drilled for countersinking flat-head wood screws that attach the bar brackets to the wooden arms (Fig. 4-36).

Mounting bolts allow you to adjust the height of bar brackets, as shown in Fig. 4-37. Two holes are drilled 6 inches apart on the lower section of the arm, as shown in Fig. 4-38. A series of holes are made 3 inches apart in the upper section. It is important to drill the holes at matching heights on the arms so that the barbell will be level when placed on the rack.

The pattern for the construction of a steel fixed-height weight stand for attachment to a

metal base is shown in Fig. 4-39. Adjustable arms are shown in Fig. 4-40. The assembly of the weight stand to the metal base is shown in Fig. 4-41. The lower end of the mounting arms form legs that add support when a barbell is placed on the rack. The parts are cut from steel pipe stock and brazed or welded together and to the metal base of the bench.

The pattern for the bar brackets is shown in Fig. 4-42. You will need two of these, one for each arm. The brackets are brazed or welded to the upper ends of the arms, as shown in Fig. 4-43.

Adjustable arms are made in two sections, as shown in Fig. 4-44. The upper section of each arm slides inside the lower section. One hole is drilled in the lower section of each mounting

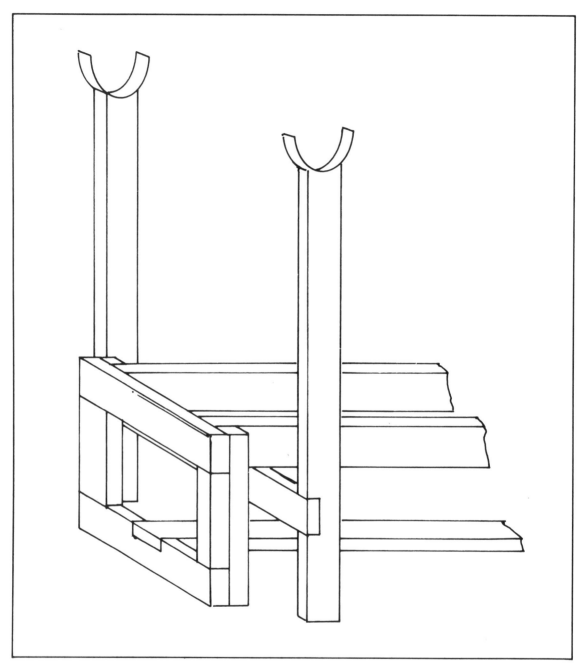

Fig. 4-32. Wood arms for bar rack at fixed height.

arm, and a series of holes 3 inches apart is drilled on the upper section. The holes for the two arms must be of the same height so that the barbell will be level when placed on the rack. Adjust-

ment bolts (one on each side) are used to hold the arms at desired height.

The basic flat weight training benches detailed above can also be constructed so that they have fixed (Fig. 4-45) or adjustable (Fig. 4-46) inclined sections. This allows additional exercises.

Inclined benches are often made longer than the basic flat bench detailed above, such as a 5-foot long bench with 18-inch flat section and 3 ½-foot inclined section (Fig. 4-47).

The hinging arrangement for the inclined section of a bench with adjustable incline is shown in Fig. 4-48. An adjusting rod that connects to weight stand arms is shown in Fig. 4-49.

Keep in mind that hundreds of variations are possible. The benches can be longer, shorter,

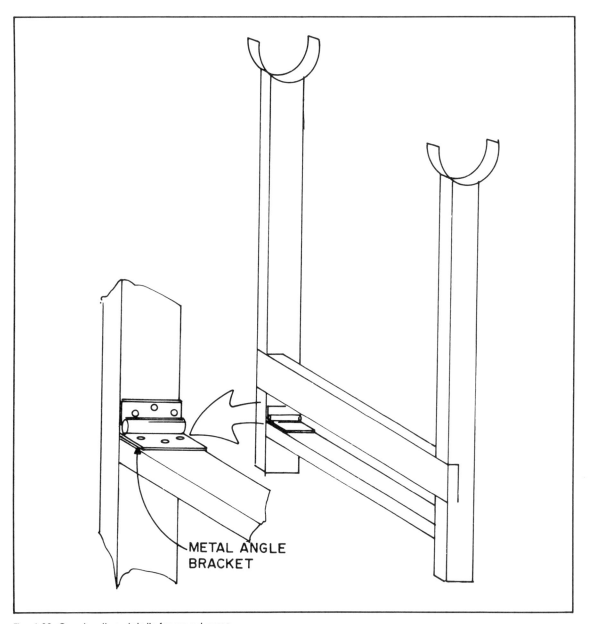

Fig. 4-33. Construction details for wood arms.

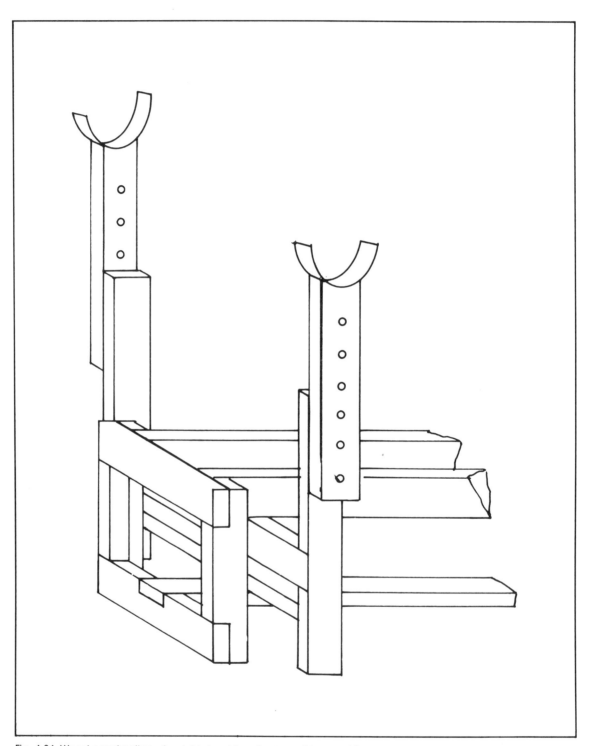

Fig. 4-34. Wood construction of weight stand for attachment to wood base.

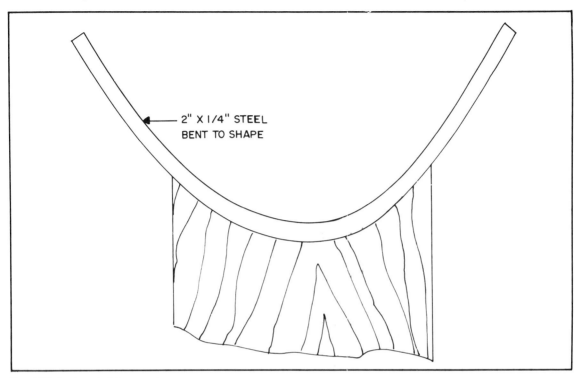

Fig. 4-35. Bar bracket for wood arm.

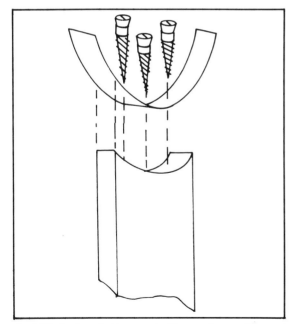

Fig. 4-36. Bar bracket is mounted to wood arm with wood screws.

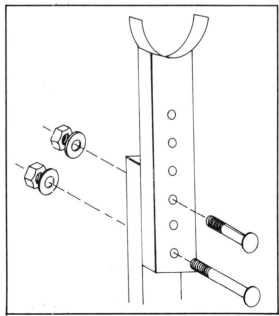

Fig. 4-37. Mounting bolts allow adjustment of height of bar bracket.

2" X 1/4" STEEL BENT TO SHAPE

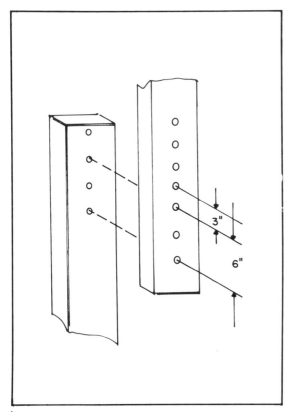

Fig. 4-38. Mounting holes for adjustable arm.

narrower, wider, lower, higher, and so on. Various inclines and even more than one incline in the same bench can be used.

SIT-UP PLATFORMS

Level or inclined sit-up platforms are popular and useful exercise devices. A platform with a fixed angle of incline is shown in Fig. 4-50. The construction details for the base are shown in Fig. 4-51. The top is cut from ½-inch plywood (Fig. 4-52).

A platform with adjustable angles of incline is shown in Fig. 4-53. The construction details for the base and platform are shown in Fig. 4-54. The construction of the top is shown in Fig. 4-55.

For both constructions, the platform is padded with foam rubber and covered with fabric backed vinyl or other suitable covering material, as shown in Fig. 4-56. The covering

material is folded around and under the wooden base and stapled or tacked in place. An adjustable web strap is used for the feet, as shown in Fig. 4-57. If desired, a foam pad can be added to the strap.

Wall bars, as detailed in Chapter 5, can be used in place of the stand for a sit-up platform with adjustable angles of incline.

STEP-UP BENCHES

Step-up benches are useful, easy-to-construct pieces of exercise equipment. The construction plan of a basic step-up bench is shown in Fig.

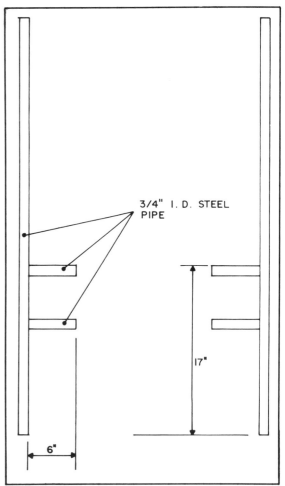

Fig. 4-39. Pattern for metal construction of fixed-height weight stand for metal base.

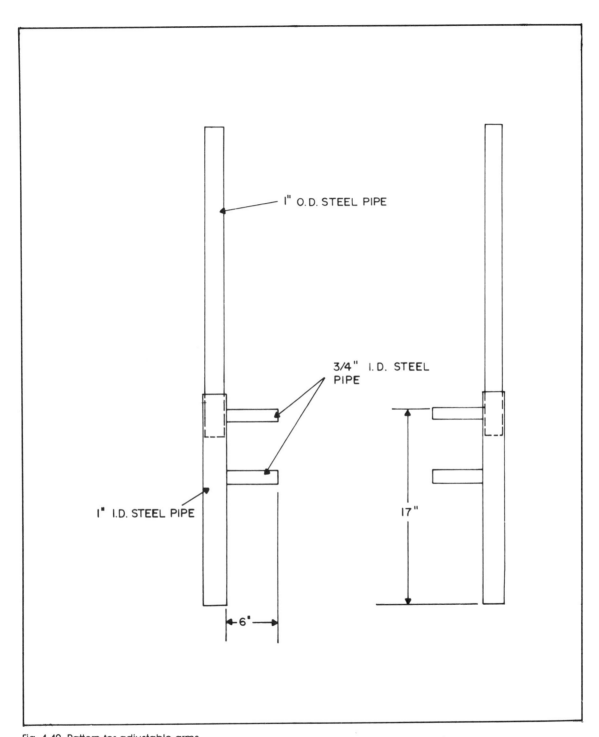

I" O.D. STEEL PIPE

3/4" I.D. STEEL PIPE

I" I.D. STEEL PIPE

17"

6"

Fig. 4-40. Pattern for adjustable arms.

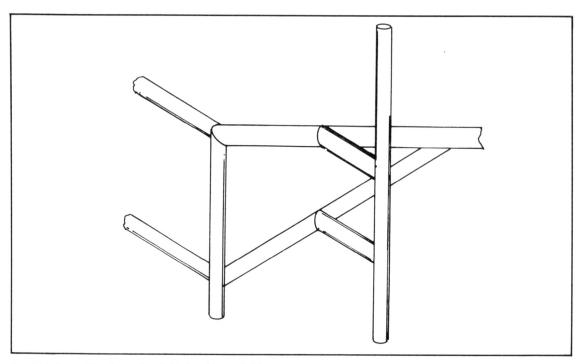

Fig. 4-41. Assembly of metal weight stand to metal base.

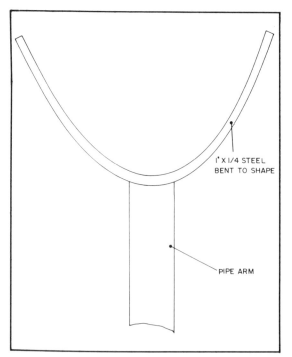

I" X I/4 STEEL
BENT TO SHAPE

PIPE ARM

Fig. 4-42. Bar bracket for pipe arm.

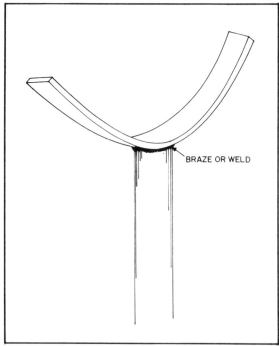

BRAZE OR WELD

Fig. 4-43. Bar bracket is brazed or welded to pipe arm.

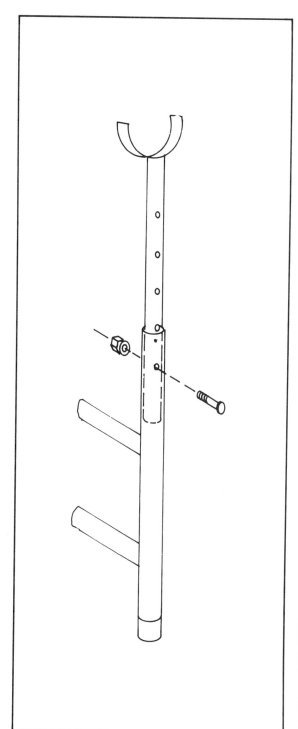

Fig. 4-44. Adjustment bolt for arm.

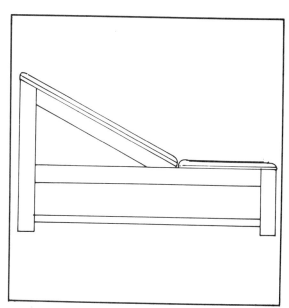

Fig. 4-45. Weight bench with fixed-angle inclined section.

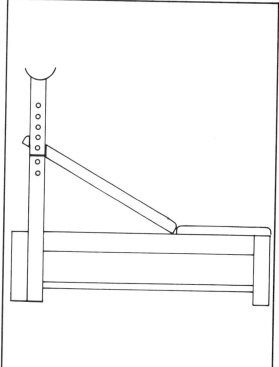

Fig. 4-46. Weight bench with adjustable inclined section.

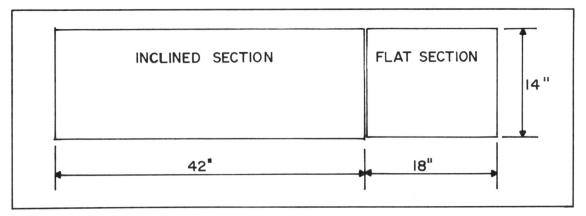

INCLINED SECTION	FLAT SECTION

14"

42"   18"

Fig. 4-47. Dimensions for inclined bench top.

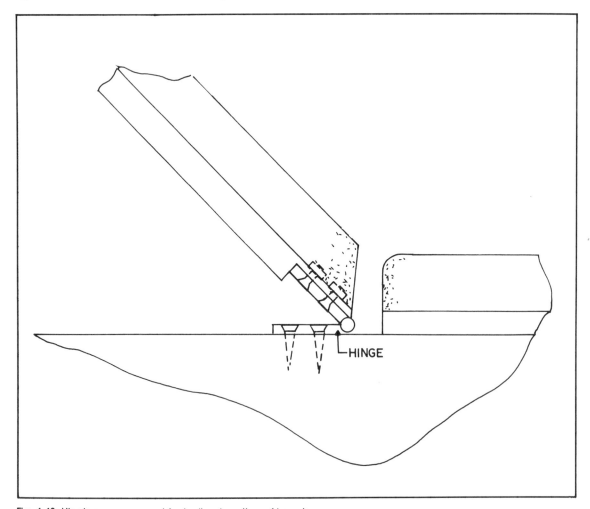

HINGE

Fig. 4-48. Hinging arrangement for inclined section of bench.

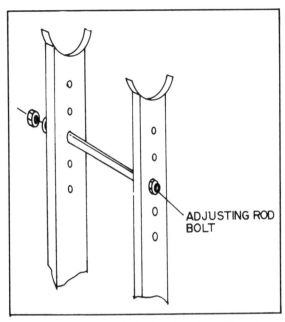

Fig. 4-49. Adjusting rod for inclined section of bench.

ADJUSTING ROD
BOLT

4-58. Assembly is by means of epoxy glue and nails.

A two-level step-up bench is shown in Fig. 4-59. You can do step-up exercise to the lower level, to the upper level, or a sequence of two steps. The construction plan is shown in Fig. 4-60. Assembly is with epoxy glue and nails.

EXERCISE MATS

Exercise mats are useful exercise equipment. While many exercises can be done on a hard floor, the mats can make them safer and more comfortable.

Exercise mats can be made by covering foam rubber or other suitable padding with canvas or plastic. If foam rubber is used, it should be firm so that it will not fully compress or "bottom out" from your weight.

The covering material can be sewn in a simple sack pattern, as shown in Fig. 4-61, or you can use the slightly more difficult box pattern, as shown in Fig. 4-62. The sewing is best

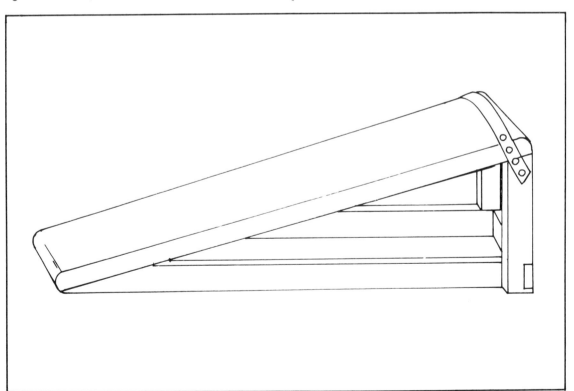

Fig. 4-50. Inclined sit-up platform with fixed angle of incline.

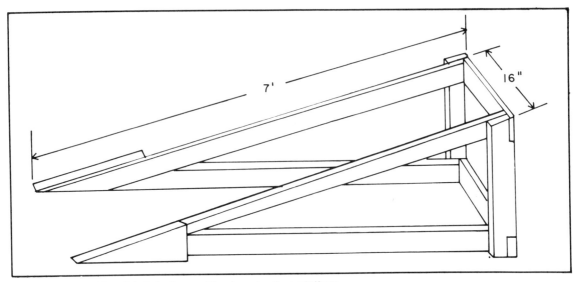

Fig. 4-51. Construction details for base of fixed-angle sit-up platform.

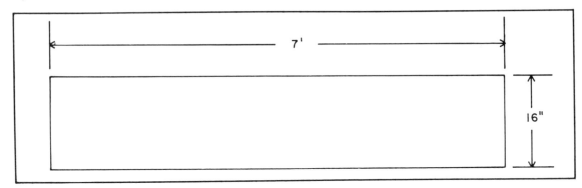

Fig. 4-52. Top is cut from ½-inch plywood to pattern shown.

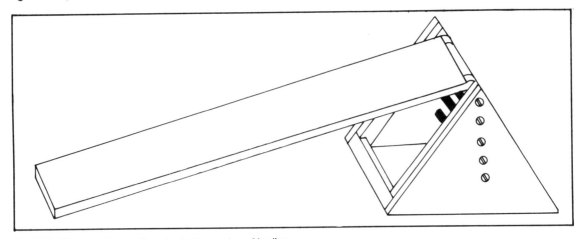

Fig. 4-53. Sit-up platform with adjustable angles of incline.

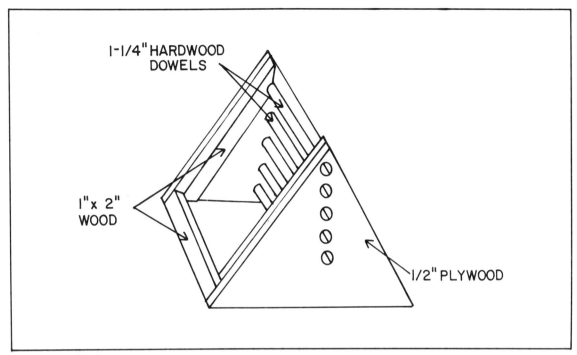

Fig. 4-54. Construction details for base of adjustable sit-up platform.

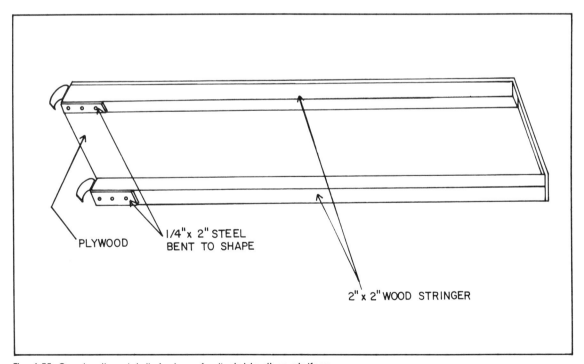

Fig. 4-55. Construction details for top of adjustable sit-up platform.

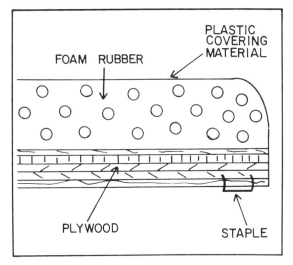

Fig. 4-56. Padded top for sit-up platform.

Fig. 4-57. Foot strap for sit-up platform.

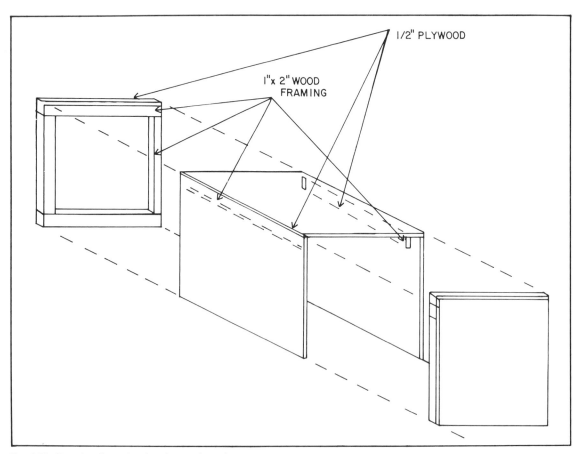

Fig. 4-58. Construction plan for step-up bench.

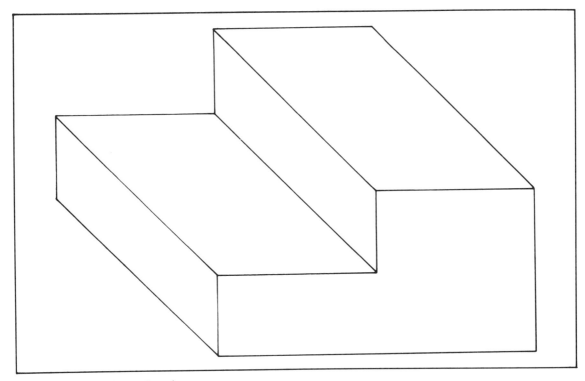

Fig. 4-59. Two-level step-up bench.

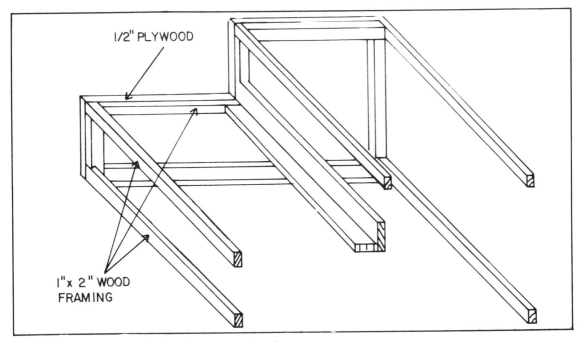

1/2" PLYWOOD

1"x 2" WOOD
FRAMING

Fig. 4-60. Construction plan for two-level step-up bench.

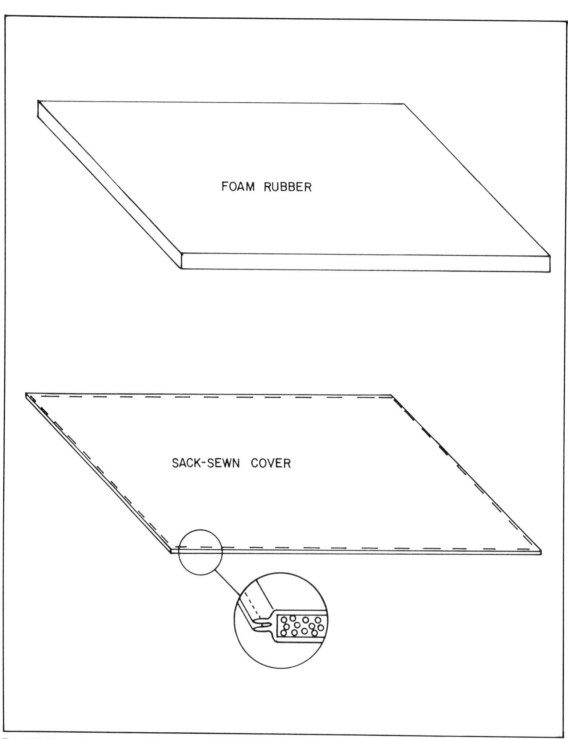

FOAM RUBBER

SACK-SEWN COVER

Fig. 4-61. Exercise mat with sack-sewn cover.

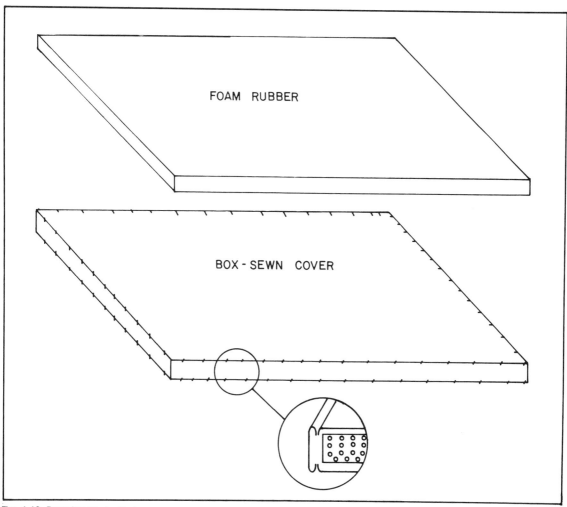

FOAM RUBBER

BOX - SEWN COVER

Fig. 4-62. Exercise mat with box-sewn cover.

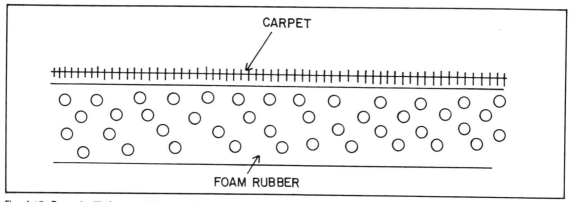

CARPET

FOAM RUBBER

Fig. 4-63. Carpet with foam rubber pad.

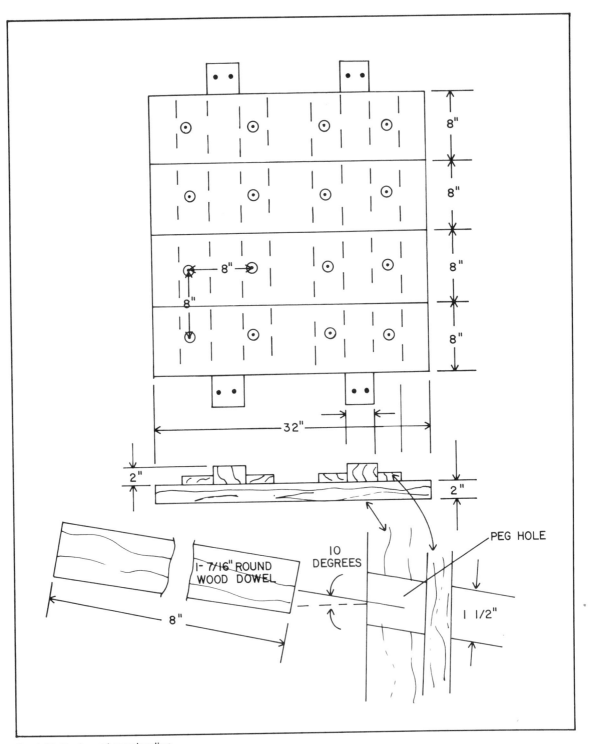

Fig. 4-64. Pegboard construction.

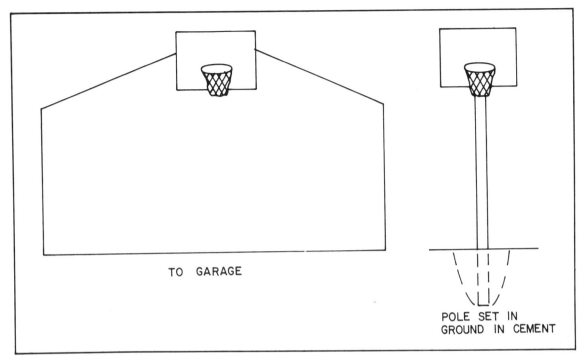

TO GARAGE

POLE SET IN
GROUND IN CEMENT

Fig. 4-65. Basketball backboard mountings.

done by machine, although hand sewing can be used if desired.

The exercise mats can be made to any desired size and thickness. This will depend on the available padding materials, the type of exercises you intend to do, amount of space available, and so on.

An alternate method is to place carpet over a foam rubber pad, as shown in Fig. 4-63. This can be free-standing if fairly stiff, heavy carpet material is used, or you can inlay the carpet over the foam padding in the exercise area or entire room, attaching it around the edges with standard carpet attachment strips.

PEG BOARD

The construction of a pegboard is shown in Fig. 4-64. The wall frame is constructed from 2×8, 2×4, and 1×4 wood stock, as shown. The 1-½-inch diameter peg holes are spaced 8 inches apart. The holes angle upward at a 10-degree angle. The wall frame should be securely mounted to a wall. If possible, through-bolts should be used.

Two wooden hand dowels 8 inches long and 1 $^7/_{16}$-inch in diameter are used. The basic exercise is to hold the pegs in your hands and climb upward, downward, and sideways by switching the pegs from hole to hole.

BASKETBALL BACKBOARDS

Setting up home basketball backboards is another possibility. You can purchase backboards made from wood or metal, or you can use plywood and cut your own to shape. The backboards can be mounted to a garage or to a pole set in cement in the ground, as shown in Fig. 4-65.

While backboards are sometimes mounted flush with a wall or post, this does present a safety hazard. It is much better to use extension arms or frame so that the backboard is about 3 feet or more from the wall or post. A sturdy mounting frame is required.

Chapter 5

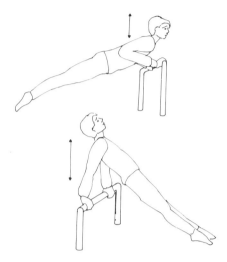

Bars and Balance Beams

Some of the plans and instructions for exercise bars and balance beams are for free-standing equipment in the sense that no floor, wall, or ceiling attachments are required and nothing is set down in the ground. Other items require floor, wall, or ceiling attachment or are set into the ground. With other items, you will have a choice of making them free standing or mounted.

HORIZONTAL OR CHINNING BARS

Horizontal or chinning bars (Fig. 5-1) are used for chin-ups and other exercises where you use your own body weight as the resistance for the exercise. Our purpose here is to detail the construction of horizontal bars that are intended for chin-ups, leg lifts, and other similar exercises. This equipment is not intended for swinging work and gymnastics, which requires much more sophisticated equipment.

Set-in-Ground

Chin-up bars are often set in the ground, such as those used for outdoor playground equipment

and as part of outdoor exercise and circuit training courses. The posts are usually set in the ground in cement.

Figure 5-2 shows the construction of a chin-up bar with 4 × 6-inch wood posts. The bottom sections should be treated with a wood preservative before being set in cement in the ground.

A 1-inch inside diameter section of galvanized pipe that is threaded on both ends is used for the bar. The length can vary. Two feet long is about minimum for chin-ups. From 3 to 4 feet long is usually better.

Holes 1¼-inch in diameter are drilled through the posts at a horizontal level for the bar. The height of the bar will depend on how you want to use it and on how tall the people who use it are. A low bar can be used for chin-ups with your feet on the ground, as shown in Fig. 5-3. In most cases, you will want to bar at a height where you can't touch the ground with your feet when you are hanging from the bar. Depending on height and arm length, this will range from about 75 to 95 inches for most adults. Floor flanges are then threaded over the ends of the bar, as shown in Fig. 5-4, and attached to the posts

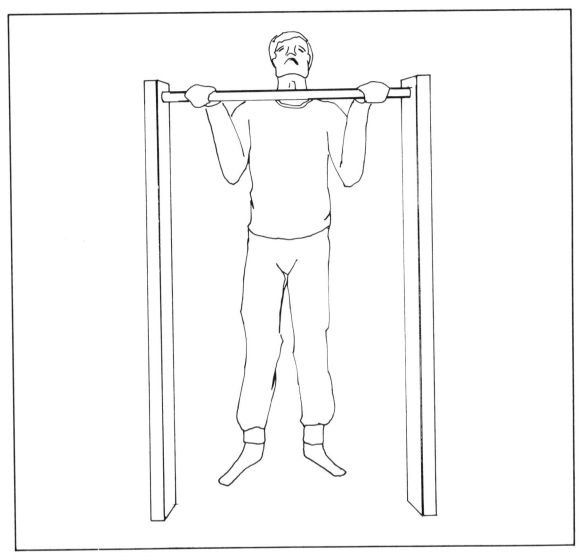

Fig. 5-1. Horizontal or chinning bar.

with wood screws. This keeps the bar from sliding out of the posts and from turning (it is very difficult to grip a bar that turns).

For the actual construction, you may want to assemble the bar to the posts first, before setting the posts in the ground. Then apply preservative to the parts of the posts that will be below the ground. The above ground section can be treated with a clear preservative or painted, either now or after the posts have been set in the ground.

Next, dig the holes for the posts. A posthole digger is handy for this, but a shovel can also be used. As a general rule, 3 feet is about minimum depth to set the posts into the ground. (The holes should be larger than the posts to allow space for the cement.)

Next, mix the cement with sand and gravel or use ready-mix cement. Add water and mix thoroughly as per the directions for the particular cement. Set up the bar in the holes and prop it in position. Check the bar with a level to make certain that it is in a horizontal position and that the posts are vertical. Allow the cement to set up before using the bar.

A similar bar can be constructed with metal posts, as shown in Fig. 5-5. In this case, the posts are made from 2-inch inside diameter galvanized pipe. Elbows with one end for the threads on the 2-inch inside diameter pipe posts and the other for the threads on the 1-inch inside diameter pipe bar are used to connect the posts to the bar.

After assembling the posts to the bar, dig the holes in the ground. A posthole digger is handy, but you can use a shovel. As a general rule, the holes should be at least 3 feet deep. Set the bar up in the holes and check it with a level to make certain that it is horizontal, and the posts are vertical.

Next, mix the cement according to the manufacturer's directions. Fill up the holes around the posts to ground level. Allow the cement to set up before using the bar.

You can also have two horizontal bars of different heights in line, as shown in Fig. 5-6, or four bars each at a different height arranged in a square, as shown in Fig. 5-7.

Freestanding

Freestanding chin-up bars are somewhat difficult to construct, as they require a large base for

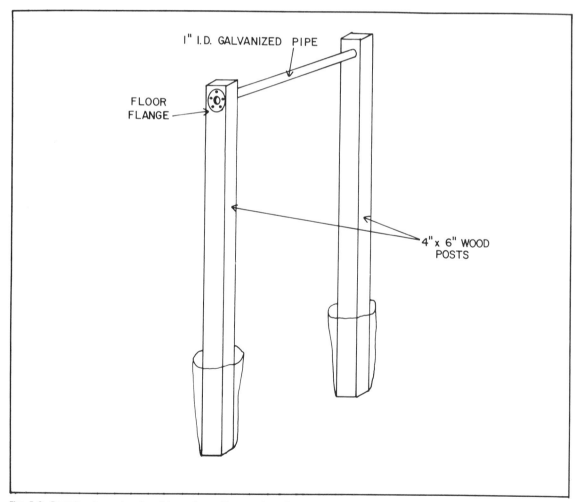

Fig. 5-2. Construction plan for chin-up bar with wood posts.

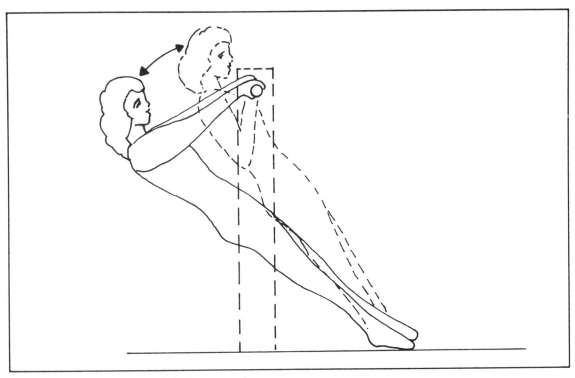

Fig. 5-3. Low bar for chin-ups with feet on ground.

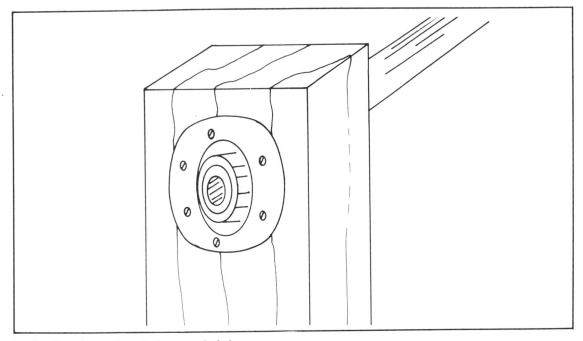

Fig. 5-4. Floor flange threaded over end of pipe.

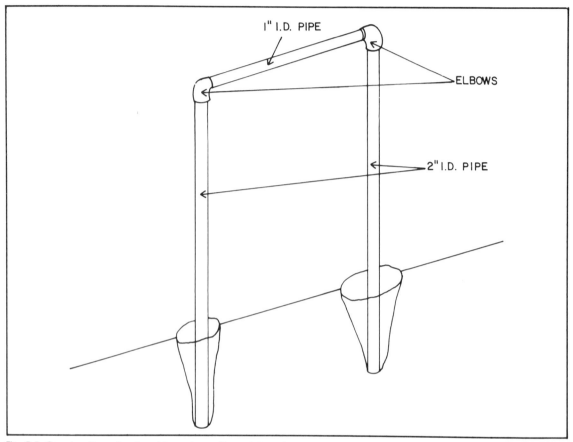

Fig. 5-5. Construction plan for chin-up bar with metal posts.

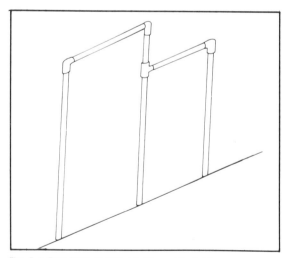

Fig. 5-6. Two bars in line at different heights.

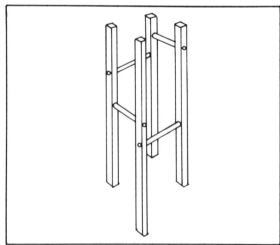

Fig. 5-7. Four bars each at different height arranged in a square.

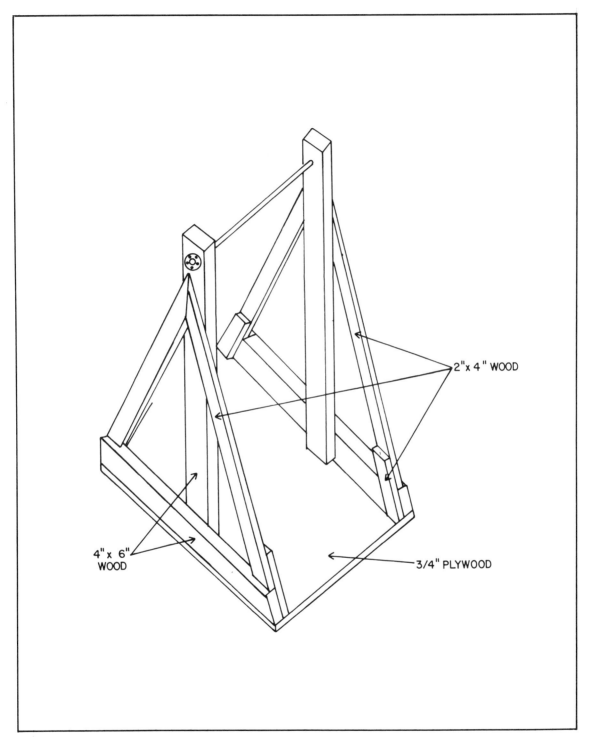

2"x 4" WOOD

4"x 6"
WOOD

3/4" PLYWOOD

Fig. 5-8. Freestanding chin-up bar.

adequate support. A design based on two 4 × 6-inch wooden beams is shown in Fig. 5-8.

Another possibility is to make the chin-up bar part of a weight bench assembly, as shown in Fig. 5-9. In this case, the bench and the chin-up bar share a common base.

Floor, Wall, and Ceiling Attachments

Chin-up bars are sometimes mounted to floors, walls, and ceilings. These methods are frequently used for "built-in" home exercise rooms. A mounting in a wooden floor is shown in Fig. 5-10. Figure 5-11 shows a combination floor and wall mounting. A wall mounting is shown in Fig. 5-12. Figure 5-13 shows a combination wall and ceiling attachment. A hanging ceiling attachment is shown in Fig. 5-14. In each case, it will be necessary to have suitable floors, walls, and/or ceilings to make these attachments. Beams for attachments must be both

suitably located and strong. Whenever possible, use through-bolts to mount fasteners. When this is not possible, lag bolts may suffice if enough of them are used, and they are properly installed in strong wooden beams.

A major disadvantage to floor, wall, and ceiling attachments is that you must make holes for fasteners. Make certain that this will not damage the building structure. I know of one person, for example, who tried to connect a tightwire to the side of a garage. He used a large eye bolt, which he through-bolted to a 2 × 4-inch framing wood in the garage wall. When he started to tighten up the wire cable, however, he almost pulled the side out of the garage. While the stresses are often less from chin-up bars, the same type of things can happen. In some cases, it will be necessary to reinforce floors, walls, and ceilings to make them suitable for mounting chin-up bars.

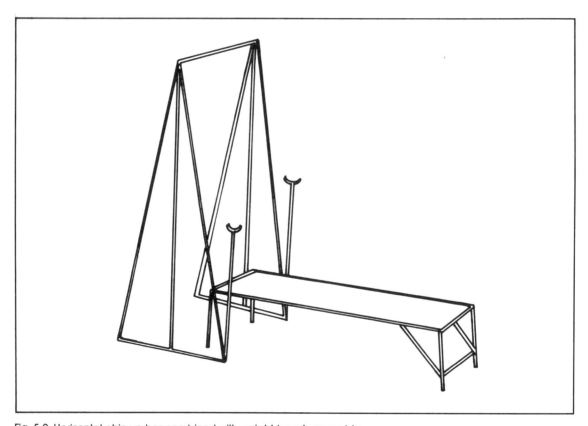

Fig. 5-9. Horizontal chin-up bar combined with weight bench assembly.

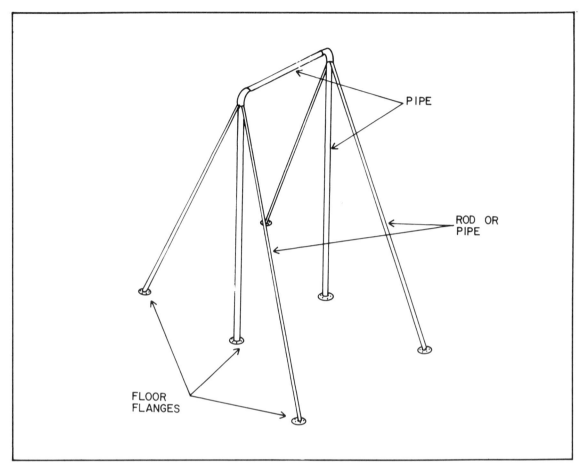

Fig. 5-10. Floor mounted chin-up bar.

PARALLEL OR DIPPING BARS

Two bars about 2 feet apart are useful for dipping (Fig. 5-15), hand walking, and other exercises. While parallel bars are also used in gymnastics competition, the bars detailed here are intended only for dipping, hand walking, and other similar exercises, and not for swinging gymnastic-type work, which require more sophisticated equipment.

Set-In-Ground

Parallel or dipping bars can be set up outdoors in the ground. Galvanized pipe can be used, and the bars can be larger diameter than for a chinning bar, because you will be supporting your weight above the bars rather than hanging from the bar, as is the case for chin-ups. Pipe with 1½-inch to 2-inch outside diameter works well for parallel bars.

If you only intend to do dipping exercises, the bars do not need to be very long—3 feet will suffice for this. For hand walking and other similar exercises, 5 or 6 feet, or longer, work well.

The height above the ground depends on the type of exercises that will be done and who will be doing them. For dipping, from 5 to 5½ feet above the ground is about right for most adults. This will also serve for hand walking and other similar exercises.

If wooden posts are used, 4 × 4-inch is about the minimum size for adequate strength. The pipe bars are threaded on both ends. Holes are drilled to pass the bars through the posts, as

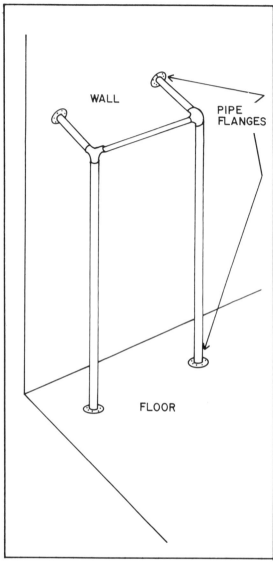

WALL

PIPE
FLANGES

FLOOR

Fig. 5-11. Combination floor and wall mounting of chin-up bar.

shovel can also be used. The holes should be larger than the posts to allow space for cement. Before placing the posts in the holes, the part that will be below the ground should be treated with a wood preservative. The part of the posts that will be above the ground can be treated with a clear preservative or painted, either now or after the posts have been set in the ground.

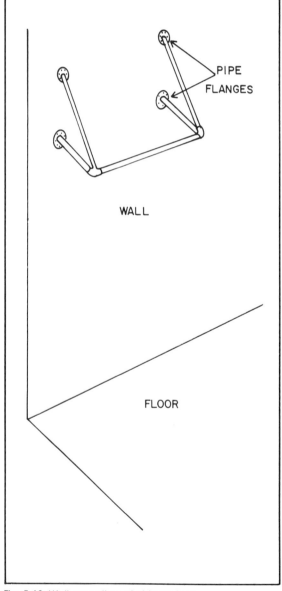

PIPE
FLANGES

WALL

FLOOR

Fig. 5-12. Wall mounting of chin-up bar.

shown in Fig. 5-16. Floor flanges are then threaded over the ends of the pipes and attached to the posts with wood screws. This will keep the pipe bars from slipping out of the posts and from turning.

The posts are set in cement filled holes. As a general rule, 3 feet is about the minimum depth that will give adequate strength. A posthole digger is handy for making the holes, but a

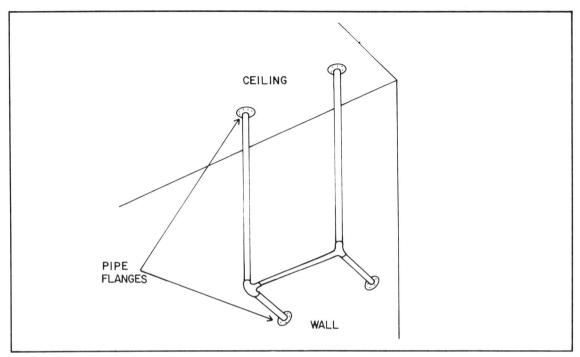

Fig. 5-13. Wall and ceiling mounting of chin-up bar.

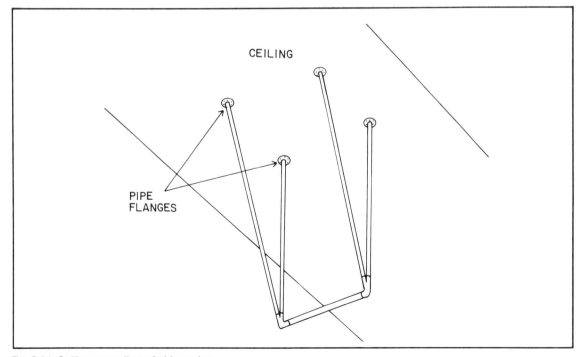

Fig. 5-14. Ceiling mounting of chin-up bar.

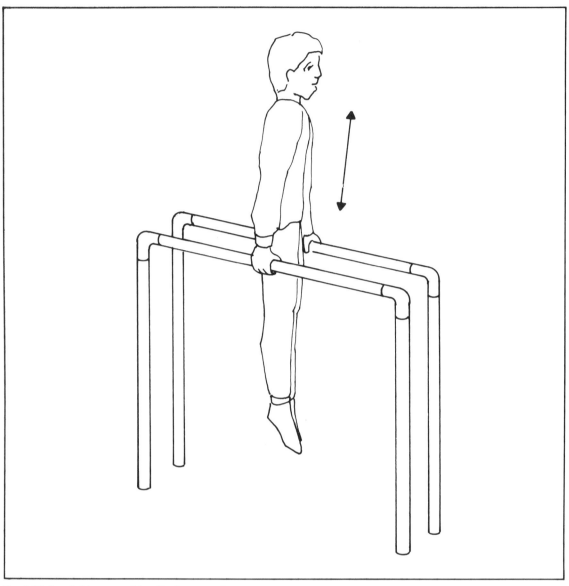

Fig. 5-15. Parallel bars used for dipping exercise.

Set up the bars in the holes and prop them in position. Check the bars to make certain that they are parallel, at the desired height, and horizontal. When everything is ready, mix the cement. Add sand and gravel to the cement or use ready-mix. Add water and mix according to the manufacturer's directions. Add the cement to the holes and fill to ground level. Allow the cement to set up before using the bars.

Parallel bars can also be constructed using metal posts, as shown in Fig. 5-17. In this case, both the posts and the bars can be made of 2-inch inside diameter galvanized pipe. Elbows are used to join the posts to the bars.

After assembly, dig the four holes in the ground with a posthole digger or a shovel. As a general rule, the holes should be at least 3 feet deep. Set the bars up in the holes and prop in

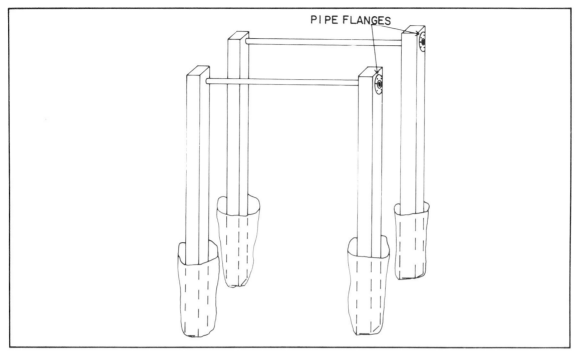

Fig. 5-16. Construction plan for parallel bars with wooden posts.

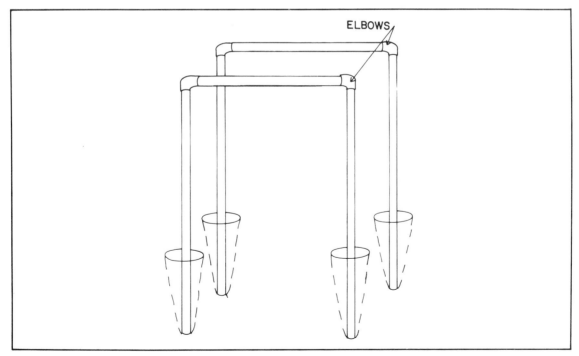

Fig. 5-17. Construction plan for parallel bars with metal posts.

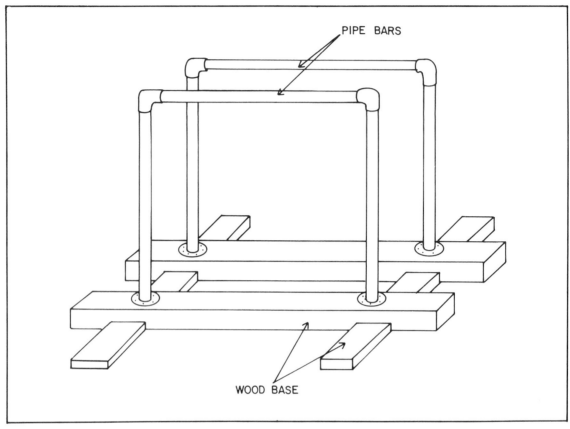

Fig. 5-18. Freestanding parallel bars.

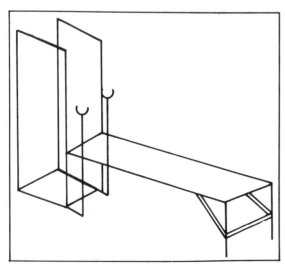

Fig. 5-19. Parallel dipping bars combined with weight bench assembly.

position; check to make certain that the bars are parallel to each other, at the same height, and horizontal, and when everything is ready, mix the cement according to the manufacturer's directions and fill up the holes around the posts to ground level. Allow the cement to set up before using the bar.

Freestanding

Freestanding parallel bars are somewhat difficult to construct, as they require a large base to give them adequate support. One possible design is shown in Fig. 5-18.

Another possibility is to make the parallel bars part of a weight bench assembly, as shown in Fig. 5-19. In this case, the bench and the parallel bars share a common base. The parallel bars are usually made quite short with this arrangement.

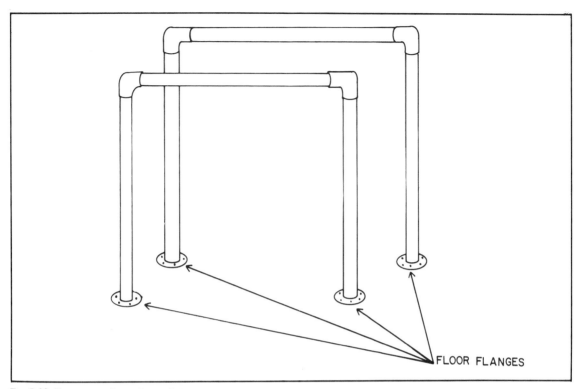

Fig. 5-20. Floor mounting of parallel bars.

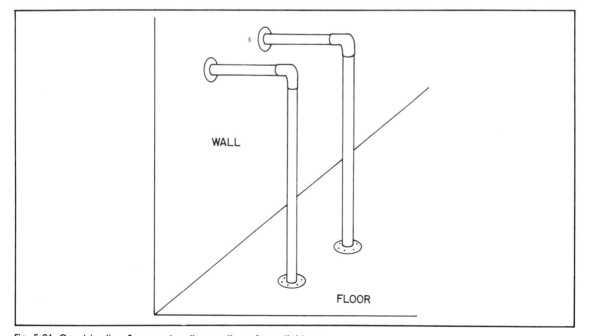

Fig. 5-21. Combination floor and wall mounting of parallel bars.

Floor and Wall Attachments

Parallel bars are sometimes mounted to floors and/or walls. These methods are frequently used for "built-in" home exercise rooms.

A floor mounting for a wooden floor is shown in Fig. 5-20. A combination floor and wall mounting is shown in Fig. 5-21. Figure 5-22 shows a wall mounting. In each case, it will be necessary to have suitable floors and/or walls. Attachment beams must be both suitably located and strong. Whenever possible, use through-bolts to mount fasteners. When this is not possible, lag bolts may suffice if enough of them are used, and they are properly installed in strong wooden beams.

WALL BARS

A series of horizontal bars placed one above the other and spaced a short distance apart outward from a wall (Fig. 5-23) make a variety of exercises possible. These bars are usually mounted to walls. They can also form the basis for pulley exercise equipment attachments, as detailed in Chapter 6.

Even a single bar at about waist height can be used for stretching exercises, such as shown in Fig. 5-24. The construction of a single wall bar from 1¼-inch inside diameter pipe is shown in Fig. 5-25. This should be attached to sturdy wall beams, preferably with through-bolts.

The construction plan for a wall unit with a

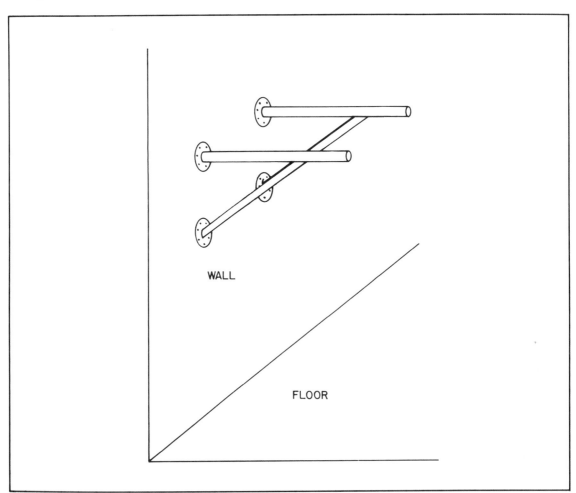

Fig. 5-22. Wall mounting of parallel bars.

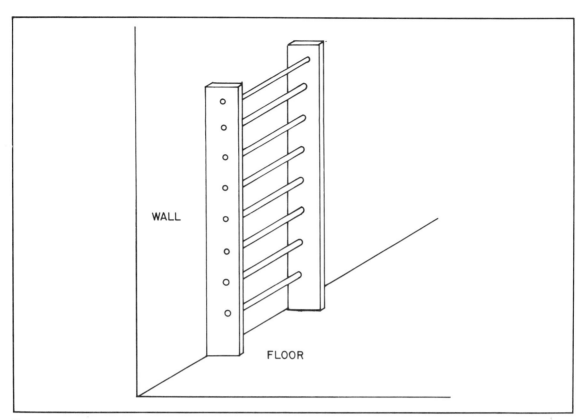

Fig. 5-23. Wall bars.

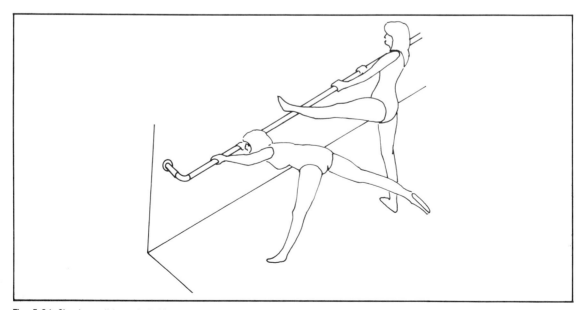

Fig. 5-24. Single wall bar stretching exercise.

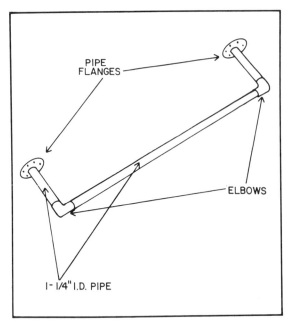

Fig. 5-25. Construction plan for single wall bar.

piece and through-bolted to the side piece. Bolts pass through this same member for mounting to the wall.

Wall bars can be left as natural wood, varnished, or painted, as desired. The bars themselves are generally best left as natural wood.

Wall bars will also serve as a stand for the adjustable sit-up platform detailed in Chapter 4, as shown in Fig. 5-29.

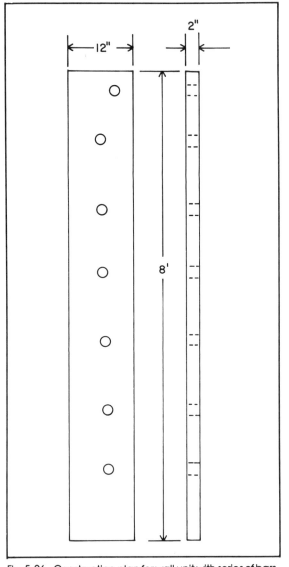

Fig. 5-26. Construction plan for wall unit with series of bars.

series of bars is shown in Fig. 5-26. The side pieces are 2 × 12-inch wood. The bars are hardwood dowels, 1½-inches in diameter. The bars can be located and spaced as desired. Spacing the bars 6 inches to 9 foot apart is typical. The number of bars can also vary. The upper bar is often placed so that your feet cannot reach the floor when you grip it and hang from it. About 93 inches from the floor will give the necessary distance for most adults. The upper bar is sometimes positioned 2 or 3 inches further outward than the lower bars for leg lifts.

Holes for the hardwood dowels are drilled in the side pieces, and the dowels are epoxy glued in place so that they will not slip out of the holes or turn.

Various types of mounting brackets can be used to bolt the unit to wall beams. One method uses steel angle pieces, as shown in Fig. 5-27. A long angle piece or series of short angle pieces can be used on each side piece. One side of the angle is through-bolted to the side piece. The other side is used to bolt the unit to the wall beams.

Another method for mounting the wall bars is to use wooden members, as shown in Fig. 5-28. A full-length piece of wood is used on each side

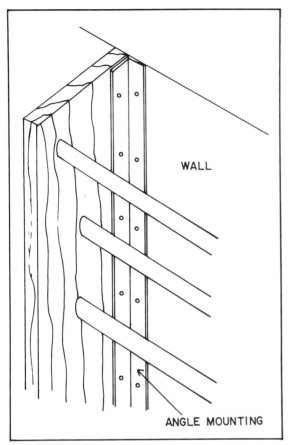

WALL

ANGLE MOUNTING

Fig. 5-27. Metal angle pieces used for wall mounting.

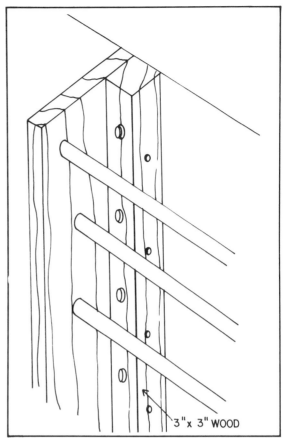

3"x 3" WOOD

Fig. 5-28. Wood member used for wall attachment bolts.

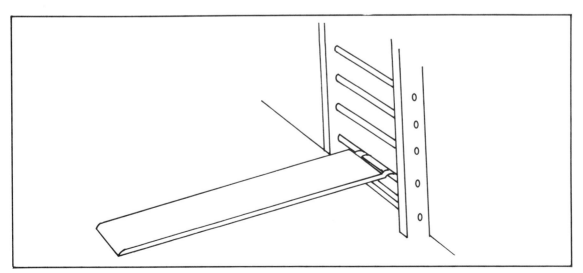

Fig. 5-29. Wall bars used as stand for adjustable sit-up platform.

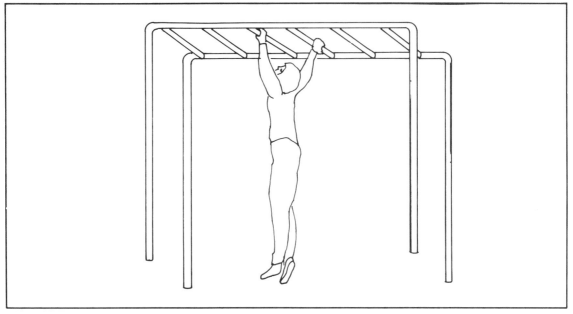

Fig. 5-30. Horizontal ladder used for overhead hand walking.

HORIZONTAL LADDERS

Horizontal ladders can be used for overhead hand walking (Fig. 5-30) and other exercises. The device is essentially a ladder with round rungs mounted in an overhead position, usually at a height that does not allow the feet to touch the ground when hanging from the bar. Horizontal ladders are popular playground devices, but they also can be used by adults for exercise purposes. They are frequently included as stations in circuit training courses. They can be constructed for home exercise either for outdoor or indoor use.

Set-in-Ground

Horizontal ladders can be set up outdoors in the ground. Steel pipe can be used to construct the ladder, the two side members can be 2-inch outside diameter steel pipe, and the rungs 1¼-inch outside diameter pipe. The rungs are brazed or welded to the side members.

Figure 5-31 shows the construction plan for mounting the ladder in the ground with 4 × 4-inch wooden posts. In this case, the ends of the side pieces of pipe are threaded on both ends. The pipes are passed through holes in the posts.

Pipe flanges are threaded on these and then attached to the wood with wood screws. This will prevent the pipes from sliding out, of the holes.

The ladder is usually mounted at a height above the ground that will allow you to hang from the bars without your feet touching the ground. This will usually vary from about 85 to 95 inches, depending on the height and arm length of the person or persons using the device.

The posts are set in the ground in cement. As a general rule, 3 feet is about the minimum depth that will give adequate strength. A post-hole digger is handy for making the holes in the ground, or a shovel can be used. The holes should be larger than the posts to allow space for cement around the posts. Before placing the posts in the holes, the sections that will be below the ground should be treated with a wood preservative. The above ground part of the posts can be treated with a clear wood preservative or painted, either at this time or later after the posts have been set in the cement.

Set the posts with the mounted ladder in the holes and prop them in position. Check to make certain that the ladder is horizontal and at the desired height. When everything is ready, mix

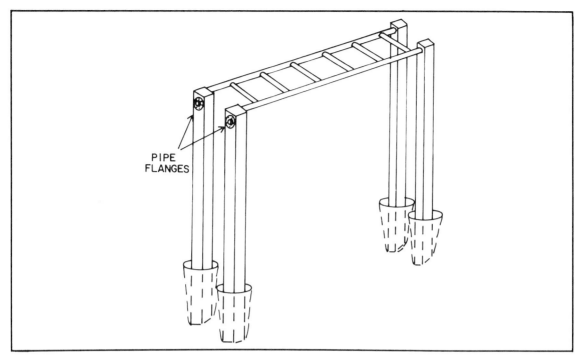

Fig. 5-31. Construction plan for horizontal ladder with wood posts.

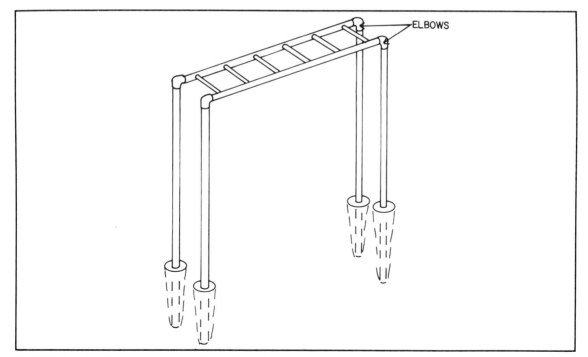

Fig. 5-32. Construction plan for horizontal ladder with metal posts.

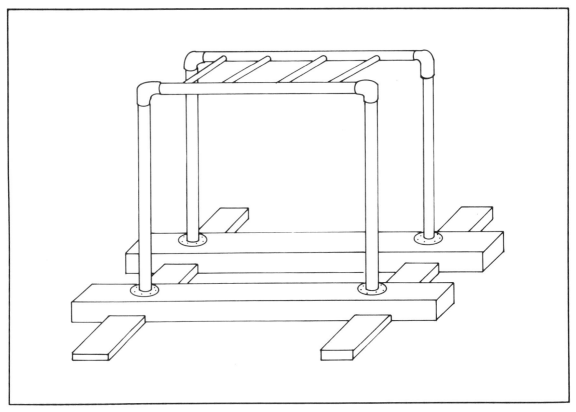

Fig. 5-33. Freestanding horizontal ladder.

the cement. Add sand and gravel to the cement or use ready-mix. Add water and mix according to the manufacturer's directions. Add the mixture to the holes and fill to ground level. Allow the cement to set up before using the horizontal ladder.

The horizontal ladder can also be constructed with metal pipe posts, as shown in Fig. 5-32. The ladder assembly is the same as for the wooden posts. Pipe elbows are threaded on the ends of the side pipes on the ladder; the pipe posts are connected to the opposite ends of the elbows.

After assembly, dig the four holes in the ground. As a general rule, the holes should be at least three feet deep. Set the assembly up in the holes and prop in position. Check to make certain that the ladder is horizontal and at the desired height above the ground. When everything is ready, mix the cement according to the manufacturer's directions and fill up the holes

around the posts to ground level. Allow the cement to set up before using the horizontal ladder.

Freestanding

Freestanding ladders can be constructed in a manner similar to the freestanding parallel bars detailed above, except that the ladder rungs are added to the parallel bars, and the bars are positioned higher from the floor (Fig. 5-33).

Floor, Wall, and Ceiling Attachments

Horizontal ladders are sometimes mounted to floors, walls, and/or ceilings. The practicality for doing this depends on the structure of the room or building where the horizontal ladder is to be installed.

A floor mounting for a wooden floor is shown in Fig. 5-34. A combination floor and

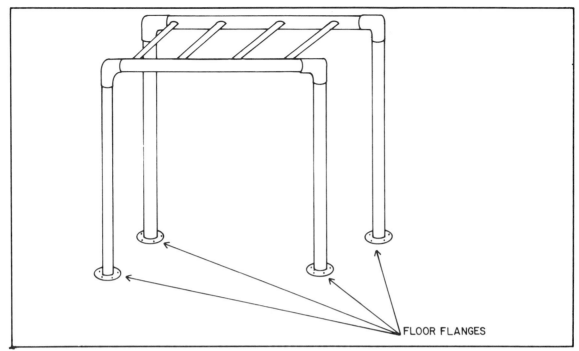

FLOOR FLANGES

Fig. 5-34. Floor mounting of horizontal ladder.

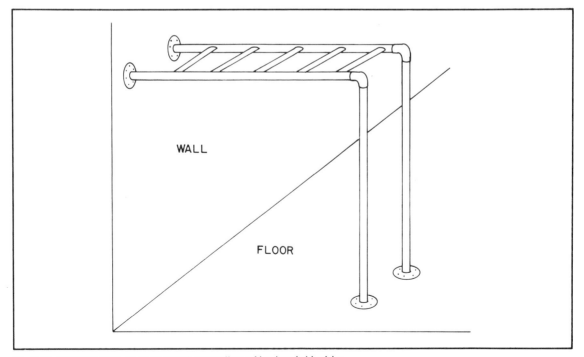

WALL

FLOOR

Fig. 5-35. Combination floor and wall mounting of horizontal ladder.

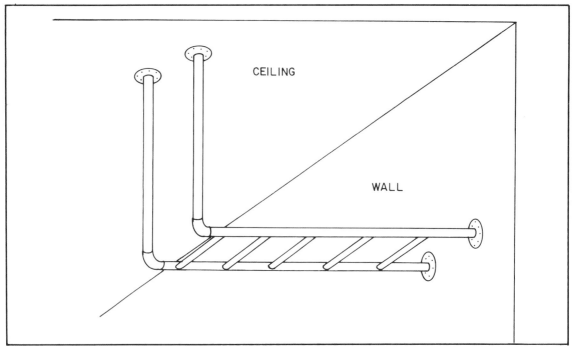

Fig. 5-36. Combination wall and ceiling mounting of horizontal ladder.

wall mounting is shown in Fig. 5-35. A combination wall and ceiling mounting is shown in Fig. 5-36. Figure 5-37 shows a ceiling mounting. In each case, it will be necessary to have suitable floors, walls, and/or ceilings to make the attach-ments, or make the necessary modifications to these so that they will be suitable. Beams, for example, must be both suitable located and strong enough. Whenever possible, use through-bolts to mount fasteners.

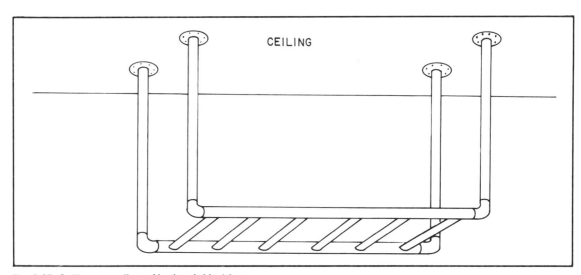

Fig. 5-37. Ceiling mounting of horizontal ladder.

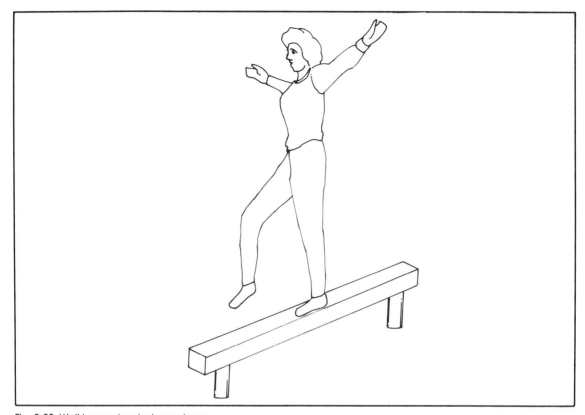

Fig. 5-38. Walking on low balance beam.

BALANCE BEAMS

Low balance beams (Fig. 5-38) are good for balance and agility exercises. The balance beams detailed here are intended only for walking and other similar exercises and not for gymnastic exercises, which require specially constructed equipment.

Set-In-Ground

Balance beams can be set in the ground, as shown in Fig. 5-39. While the height can vary, about 1 foot from the ground works well. This is high enough to perform walking exercises, yet close enough to the ground for safety. The width of the beam can also vary. Narrow widths (2

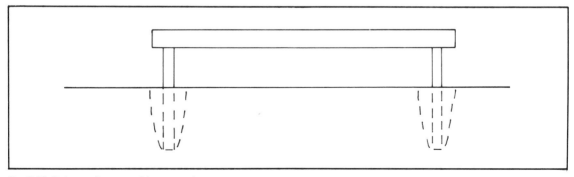

Fig. 5-39. Balance beam set in ground.

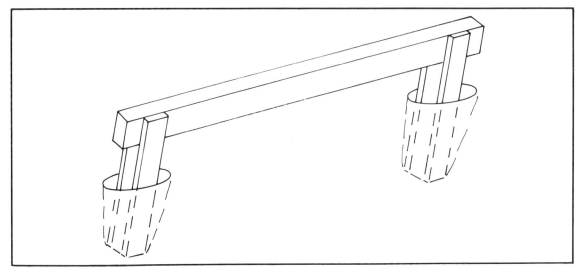

Fig. 5-40. Construction plan for wood balance beam with wood posts.

inches), are more difficult to walk than are wider widths, (up to 4 inches). The choice depends on how you intend to use the device.

The construction plan for a wooden balance beam with wooden posts is shown in Fig. 5-40. The posts should extend at least a couple of feet below ground level. Assemble the beam to the posts. Next, dig the mounting holes in the ground. The posts are set in cement in the holes. Set up the assembly in the holes and prop in position. Check the beam to make certain it is horizontal and at the desired height above the

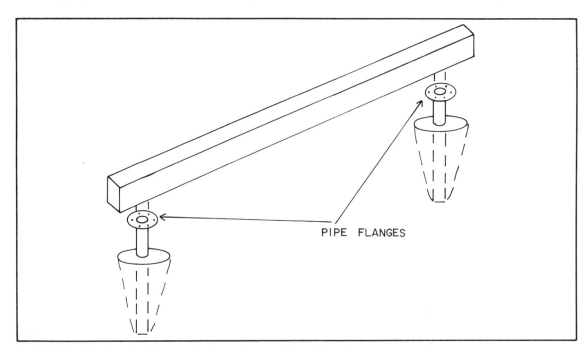

PIPE FLANGES

Fig. 5-41. Construction plan for wood balance beam with metal posts.

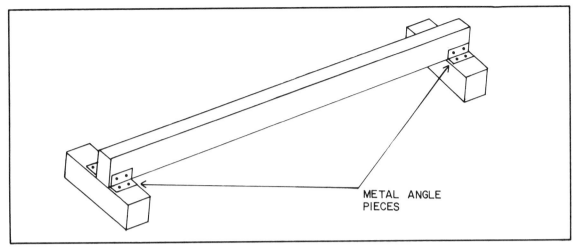

Fig. 5-42. Freestanding balance beam.

ground. When everything is ready, mix the cement with sand, gravel, and water or add water to ready-mix cement, according to manufacturer's directions. Fill holes around the posts to ground level. Allow the cement to set up before using the balance beam.

The balance beam can also be constructed using metal pipe posts, as shown in Fig. 5-41. The pipe posts are attached to the wooden beam with pipe flanges, which thread onto the ends of the pipe posts, and wood screws that attach the beam to the floor flanges.

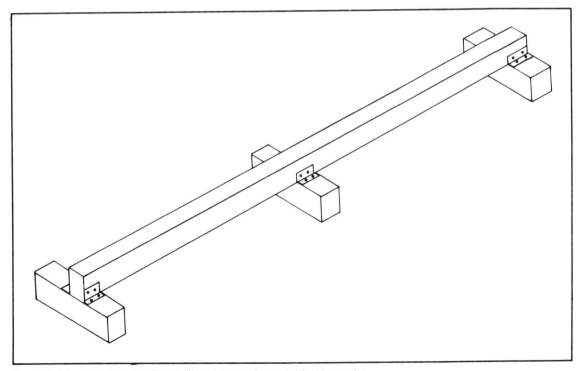

Fig. 5-43. Extra long beam with additional cross pieces added to center.

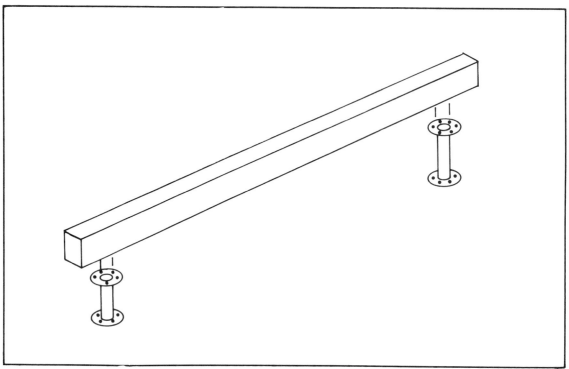

Fig. 5-44. Construction plan for floor mounted balance beam.

After assembly, dig the two holes in the ground. A posthole digger is handy for this, but a shovel can also be used. The holes should be at least a couple of feet deep. Set up the beam in the holes and prop in position. Make certain that the beam is level and at the desired height. When everything is ready, mix the cement according to the manufacturer's directions and fill up the holes around the posts to ground level. Allow the cement to set up before using the balance beam.

Freestanding

The construction plan for a freestanding balance bean is shown in Fig. 5-42. The cross pieces of wood are attached to the beam with steel angle pieces. The cross pieces should be placed at the ends of the beam so that the beam will not raise up off the floor when you stand on an end. If an extra long beam is constructed, an additional cross piece can be added to the center, as shown in Fig. 5-43.

Floor Mounting

A floor mounting for a balance beam is shown in Fig. 5-44. The pipe posts are threaded on both ends to receive the floor flanges. The upper floor flanges attach to the wooden balance beam with wood screws. The lower flanges are attached to the floor by means of through-bolts or other suitable fasteners.

PUSH-UP BARS

A push-up bar is a horizontal bar placed low to the ground. Regular push-ups (Fig. 5-45) and backward push-ups are exercises that can be done using a push-up bar. The height of the bar above the ground can vary. About 1 foot from the ground works well for many exercises, but other heights can also be used.

Set-In-Ground

Push-up bars can be set in the ground in cement. The construction plan for using wooden posts is

114

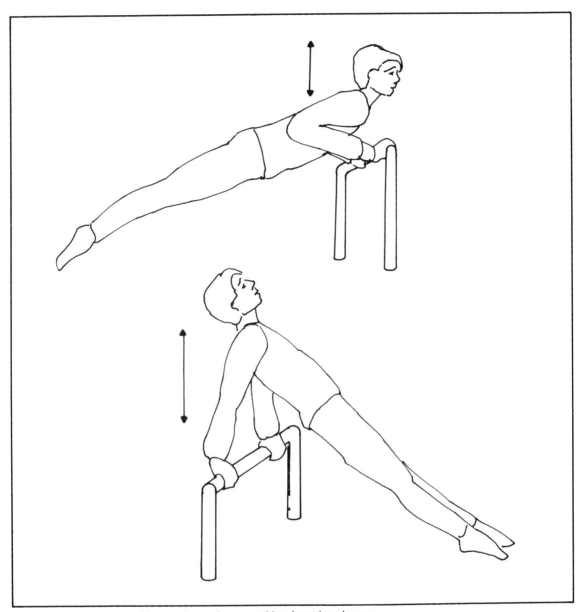

Fig. 5-45. Push-up bar used for regular push-ups and backward push-ups.

shown in Fig. 5-46. Holes are drilled in the wooden posts large enough to accept the 1¼-inch outside diameter pipe bar, which is threaded on both ends. Floor flanges are threaded onto the ends of the pipe outside the posts. The flanges are then attached to the wooden posts with wood screws.

The posts should be set in the ground at least a couple of feet. Make the holes larger than the posts to allow room for the cement fill. Sections of wood that will be below the ground should be treated with a wood preservative. Set up the bar in the holes and prop it in place. Check to make certain that the bar is level and at

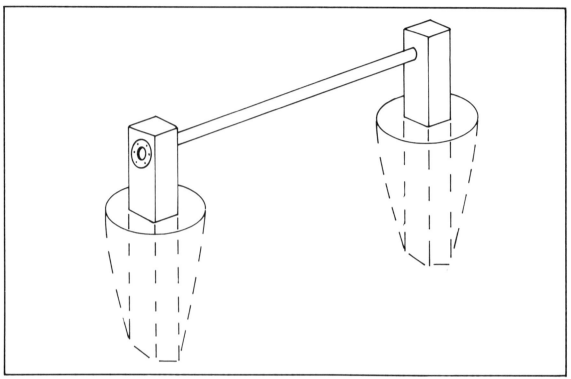

Fig. 5-46. Construction plan for push-up bar with wooden posts.

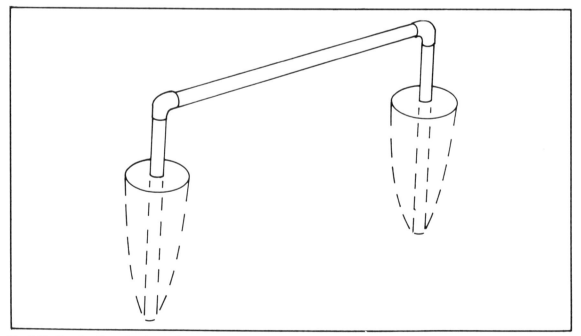

Fig. 5-47. Construction plan for push-up bar with metal posts.

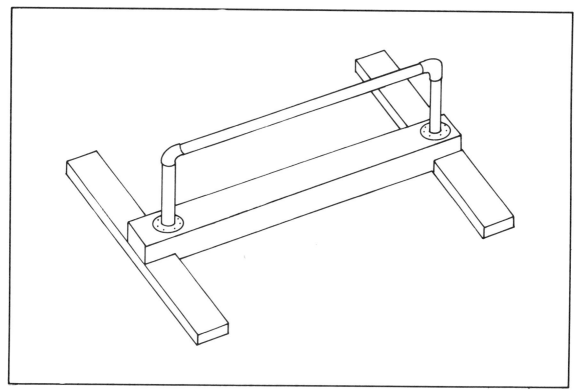

Fig. 5-48. Freestanding push-up bar.

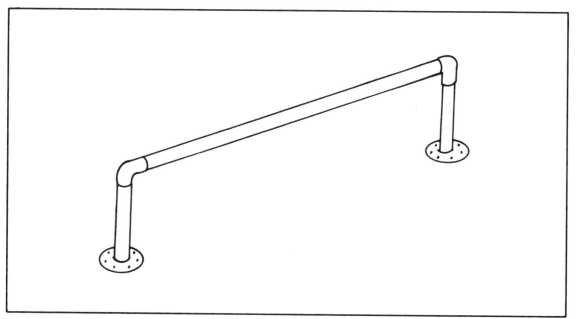

Fig. 5-49. Floor mounting of push-up bar.

117

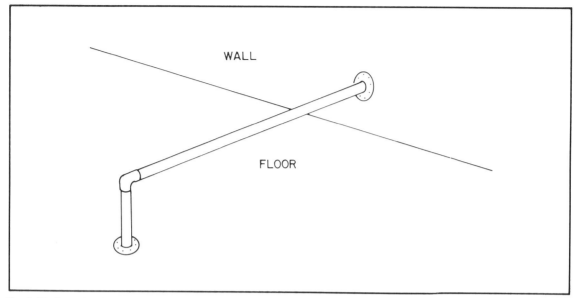

WALL

FLOOR

Fig. 5-50. Combination floor and wall mounting of push-up bar.

the desired height. When everything is ready, mix and pour the cement. Fill the holes to ground level, and allow the cement to set up before using the push-up bar.

An alternate assembly is to use pipe posts, as shown in Fig. 5-47. The posts are connected to the pipe bar with elbows, and are set in the ground in cement.

Freestanding

The construction plan for a freestanding push-up bar is shown in Fig. 5-48. The pipe posts are connected to the bar with threaded elbows. Floor flanges connect the posts to the base.

Floor and Wall Mountings

A floor mounting for a push-up bar is shown in Fig. 5-49. A combination floor and wall mounting is detailed in Fig. 5-50.

In both cases, it is important to have suitable beams to which to attach the pipe flanges with through-bolts or screws. While the stresses on low push-up bars are not nearly as great as those on chin-up bars, they can still be considerable. For this reason, it is important to use strong mountings that will not come loose when the push-up bar is being used.

Chapter 6

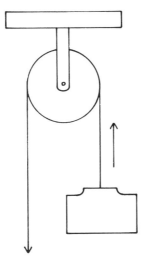

Applied Exercise Theory

BEFORE CONSTRUCTING EXERCISE EQUIPMENT, IT IS important to have a basic understanding of *simple machines*. Simple machines are devices that allow us to do work in an easier or quicker way. They permit the exertion of a force that is greater than that applied, or they change the direction of an applied force.

One type of simple machine is used to multiply a force. When you change a tire on an automobile, you cannot lift the automobile by yourself, but the use of an automobile jack allows you to do so. The jack allows a force great enough to lift the automobile when a much lesser force is exerted on the jack handle. Of course, as will be seen, you have to move the jack handle a much greater distance than the automobile is moved. Wrenches, pump handles, can openers, nutcrackers, and bottle openers are examples of other simple machines that can multiply a force. This type of simple machine is often found in exercise machines.

The purpose of some simple machines is to change the direction of an applied force. A pulley wheel can be arranged so that you can stand on the ground and raise a load upward by pulling down on a rope, as shown in Fig. 6-1. In the case of bicycling, for example, the pedals are arranged so that you can exert a downward force with your legs to move the bicycle forward. Pulley exercise machines often change the direction of an applied force so that you can do specific exercises in desired directions.

Another simple machine is used to increase the speed of and the distance covered by an applied force. The baseball bat provides an example of this. The end of the bat travels further and faster than do the hands swinging the bat. When sweeping with a broom, the hands move through a shorter distance and at a slower speed than do the bristles on the end of the broom. Other examples include golf clubs, shovels, and fishing poles, all of which increase the speed and distance covered by an applied force. This type of simple machine also has many applications in exercise devices and machines.

Regardless of how complicated, expensive, or large a machine may be, its mechanical components are made up of some combination of six fundamental, simple machines: the lever,

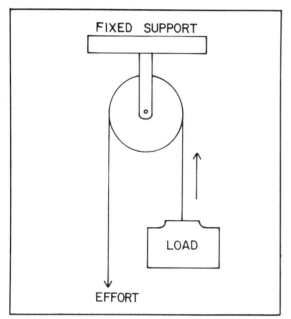

Fig. 6-1. A pulley wheel arranged to change the direction of force.

The Lever. A *lever* is a simple machine consisting of a rigid body, such as a metal bar, pivoted on a fixed fulcrum. Levers can be used to multiply a force, to gain speed or distance, or to reverse the direction of a force. We are constantly using our arms, legs, fingers, and other body segments as levers. Levers are used extensively in exercise devices and machines.

A lever has a supporting or pivoting point, called the *fulcrum* (Fig. 6-2). The lever can turn on the fixed fulcrum. The *effort* is the force that is exerted on the lever to make it turn. The *resistance* is that force which resists the effort. The force of resistance is often called the *load*. The effort and the resistance are applied at certain distances from the fulcrum. The distance between the fulcrum and the point at which the effort is applied is the *effort arm*. The distance between the fulcrum and the point at which the resistance is applied is the *resistance arm*.

The *effort moment* is the effort multiplied by the effort arm. The *resistance moment* is the resistance multiplied by the resistance arm.

A lever system is shown in Fig. 6-3. The effort moment turns the lever in a clockwise direction. The resistance moment, at the same time, turns the lever in a counterclockwise direction. When the lever is not turning (in *equilibrium*), the sum of the clockwise moments is equal to the sum of the counterclockwise moments. This is called the *law of levers*. Stated in mathematical terms, this equilibrium exists

the wheel and axle, the pulley, the inclined plane, the screw, and the wedge.

All six belong to two general classes of machines—the lever and the inclined plane.

LEVERS

Levers include the lever, the wheel and axle, and pulleys.

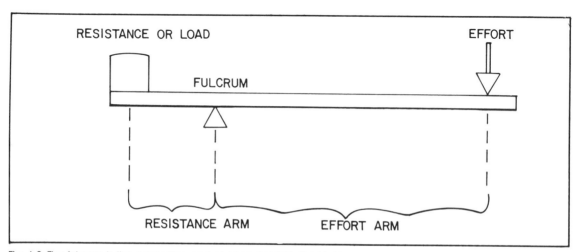

Fig. 6-2. The fulcrum is the supporting and pivoting point for the lever.

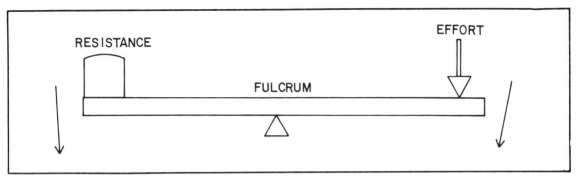

Fig. 6-3. A lever system.

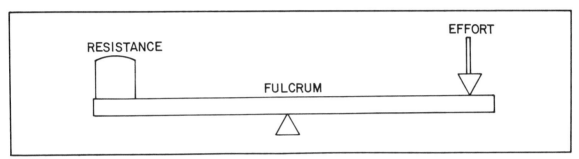

Fig. 6-4. A Class 1 lever.

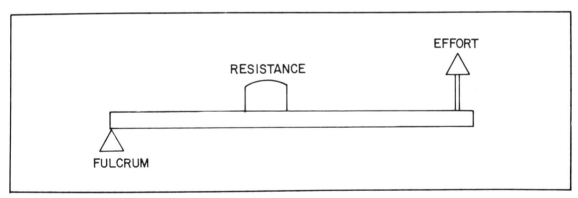

Fig. 6-5. A Class 2 lever.

when the effort moment is equal to the resistance moment, or *Effort × Effort Arm = Resistance × Resistance Arm*.

There are three classes of levers. *Class One levers* have the fulcrum between the effort moment and the resistance moment, as shown in Fig. 6-4.

A *Class Two lever* is shown in Fig. 6-5, and a *Class Three lever* in Fig. 6-6. Both of these levers have the resistance moment and the effort mo-

ment on the same side of the fulcrum. In the case of the Class Two lever, however, the resistance is closer to the fulcrum than is the effort. In the case of the Class Three lever, the effort is closer to the fulcrum than is the resistance.

A wheelbarrow, as shown in Fig. 6-7, is a common example of a Class Two lever. As a sample problem, we will determine the effort that must be applied to the handles of a wheelbarrow, which are 4 feet from the fulcrum, when

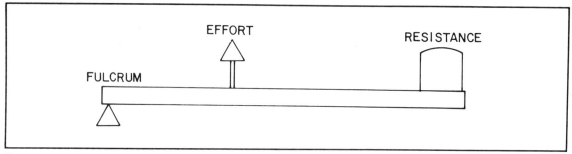

Fig. 6-6. A Class 3 lever.

the resistance (load) is 50 pounds and is concentrated at a distance of 2 feet from the fulcrum (Fig. 6-8).

The law of the lever remains the same regardless of the class of the lever. Thus, in the case of the Class Two wheelbarrow example, effort multiplied by effort arm equals resistance multiplied by resistance arm. The resistance arm is the distance from the point where the resistance arm is the distance from the point where the resistance is applied to the fulcrum, and the effort arm is the distance from the point where the effort is applied to the fulcrum. In the wheelbarrow problem, the resistance arm is equal to 2 feet. The effort arm is equal to 4 feet.

Using the law of the lever (*Effort × Effort Arm = Resistance × Resistance Arm*), we want to find out the effort that must be applied to keep the lever in equilibrium. This is equal to the resistance multipled by the resistance arm divided by the effort arm. Thus, the effort equals 50 pounds times 2 feet divided by 4 feet, which equals 25 pounds.

In order to hold the 50 pound load in equilibrium, an effort of 25 pounds must be applied to the handles of the wheelbarrow.

If we reverse the positions of the effort and resistance and use the same values as in the above example, we then have the Class Three lever shown in Fig. 6-9. Using the same formula (effort equals resistance multipled by resistance arm divided by effort arm), the effort equals 50 pounds times 4 feet divided by 2 feet, which equals 100 pounds.

In order to hold the 50 pound resistance (load) in equilibrium, an effort of 100 pounds must be applied.

The same quantities can be applied to a Class One lever. If the resistance arm is 2 feet, and the effort arm is 4 feet, as shown in Fig. 6-10,

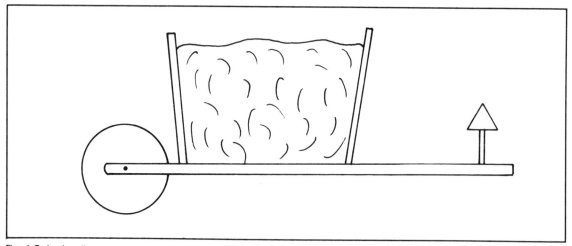

Fig. 6-7. A wheelbarrow.

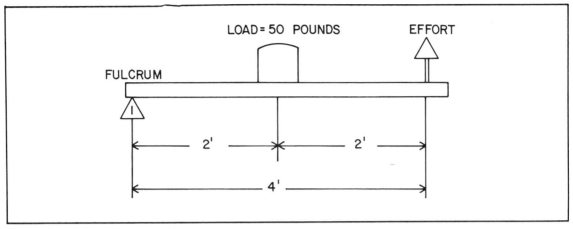

Fig. 6-8. Sample Class 2 lever problem.

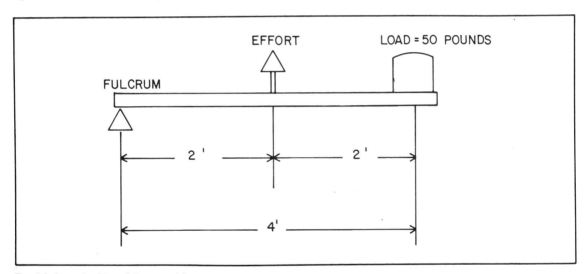

Fig. 6-9. Sample Class 3 lever problem.

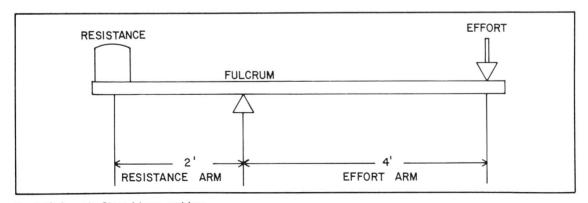

Fig. 6-10. Sample Class 1 lever problem.

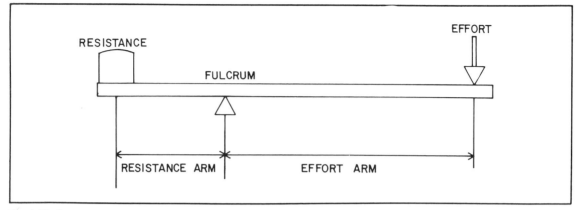

Fig. 6-11. Class 1 lever with resistance arm shorter than effort arm.

the equation is the same as for the Class Two lever example given above (effort equals resistance multipled by resistance arm divided by effort arm). If the resistance arm is 4 feet and the effort arm is 2 feet, as shown in Fig. 6-16, the equation is the same as for the Class Three lever example given above: the effort equals 50 pounds times 4 feet divided by 2 feet, which equals 100 pounds.

In the above examples, we have been concerned with a state of equilibrium. If we slightly increase the effort applied, however, the resistance will be moved, with the lever bar pivoting at the fulcrum.

There are three possibilities for a Class One lever. First, the resistance arm can be shorter than the effort arm, as shown in Fig. 6-11. In this case, the lever system changes the direction of force. Less force is required than the resistance. The force moves further and faster than the resistance.

Second, the resistance arm and the effort arm can be the same length, as shown in Fig. 6-12. In this case, the lever system changes the direction of force. The same force is required as the resistance. Both the force and resistance move the same distances and at the same rates.

Third, the resistance arm can be longer than the effort arm, as shown in Fig. 6-13. In this case, the lever system changes the direction of force. Greater force is required than resistance. The resistance moves further and faster than the force.

A Class Two lever, by definition, always has a resistance arm that is shorter than the effort arm, as shown in Fig. 6-14. In this case, the lever

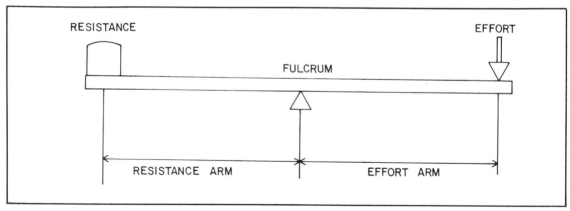

Fig. 6-12. Class 1 lever with resistance and effort arms of equal length.

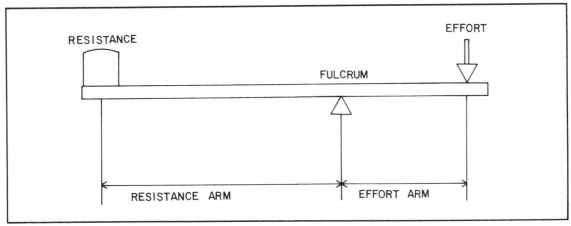

Fig. 6-13. Class 1 lever with resistance arm longer than effort arm.

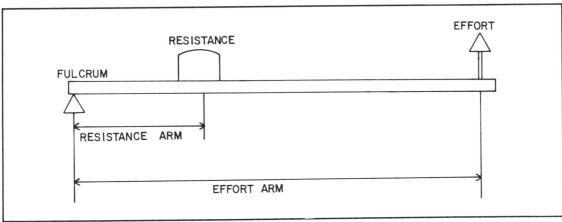

Fig. 6-14. A Class 2 lever always has a resistance arm that is shorter than the effort arm.

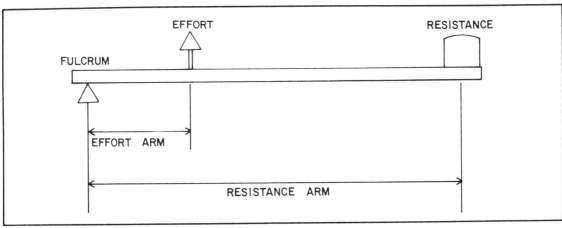

Fig. 6-15. A Class 3 lever always has a resistance arm that is longer than the effort arm.

system does not change the direction of force. If the effort is upward, the resistance also moves upward. Less force is required than the resistance; the force moves further and faster than the resistance.

A Class Three lever, by definition, always has a resistance arm that is longer than the effort arm, as shown in Fig. 6-15. In this case, the lever system does not change the direction of force. If the effort is upward, the resistance always moves upward. Greater force is required than the resistance. The resistance moves further and faster than the force.

Mechanical Advantage. Mechanical advantage is a measure of a machine's ability to assist the user, defined as the ratio of output force to the input force. In the case of the levers described above, the mechanical advantage is equal to the resistance divided by the effort. The *output force* is the resistance. The *input force* is the effort. The mechanical advantage equals the resistance divided by the effort. Mechanical advantage also equals the effort arm divided by the resistance arm. The effort arm divided by the resistance arm is equal to the resistance divided by the effort.

From this, it can be seen that the greater the difference or ratio between the length of the effort arm and the length of the resistance arm, the greater will be the difference between the resistance and the effort.

As an example, assume that we have a lever with a resistance arm that is 1 foot long and an effort arm that is 2 feet long, as shown in Fig. 6-16. It does not matter whether this is a Class One or a Class Two lever. The main difference is that in a Class One lever the direction of force changes; in a Class Two lever the direction of force does not change, but the ratios for determining mechanical advantage remain the same. If a 3-pound effort is applied, the effort arm divided by the resistance arm must have the same ratio as the resistance divided by the effort. Therefore, the resistance must be 6 pounds. The ratio for the effort arm divided by the resistance arm is two to one (2:1), and for the resistance divided by the effort is six to three (6:3). In each case, this gives a mechanical advantage of 2. Once you know this, you also know that using the same lever, you would need only a 5-pound

force of effort to overcome 10 pounds of resistance. This tells you that less force of effort is required than the resistance. For this gain, however, there must also be a sacrificed: to move the resistance a certain distance, the force of effort must move further and faster than the resistance. Force has been gained, but speed and distance have been lost. Any mechanical advantage gained, which is the difference between input and output forces, is always lost elsewhere—in this case in the distances through which these forces must act. Notice also that when the force of effort causes the lever to rotate, the resistance always moves at a slower speed than the effort. This is true regardless of the speed with which the effort moves.

As a second example, assume that we have a lever with a resistance arm that is 2 feet long and an effort arm that is 1 foot long, as shown in Fig. 6-17. It does not matter whether this is a Class One or a Class Three lever. The main difference is that in a Class One lever the direction of force changes; in a Class Three lever the direction of force does not change. The ratios for determining mechanical advantage remain the same. If a 6-pound effort is applied, then in order for the sum of the effort arm divided by the resistance arm to have the same ratio as resistance divided by effort, the resistance must be 3 pounds. The ratio for the effort arm divided by the resistance arm is 1:2 and for the resistance divided by the effort is 3:6 or 1:2. In each case, this gives a mechanical advantage of 1:2. Once you know this, you also know that using the same lever, you would need 10 pounds of force of effort to overcome 5 pounds of resistance. This tells you that more force of effort is required than the resistance. You have actually lost force, but for this sacrifice, there must also be a gain.

To move the resistance a certain distance, the force of effort moves slower and a shorter distance than the resistance. Force has been lost, but speed and distance have been gained. The mechanical advantage lost, which is the difference between input and output forces, is always made up for elsewhere, in this case in the greater distance of movement of the resistance than of the force of effort. Notice also that when the force of effort causes the lever to rotate, the resistance always moves at a faster speed than the

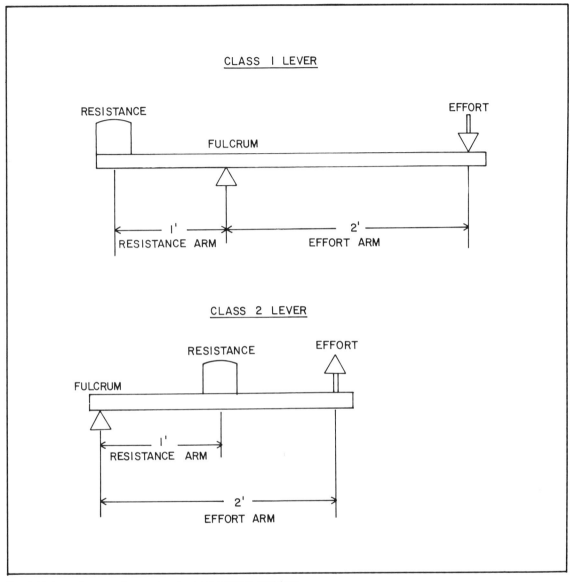

Fig. 6-16. Lever for sample mechanical advantage problem.

effort. This is true regardless of the speed with which the effort moves.

Work Done by a Lever. A machine is a mechanical device that makes use of energy to do work. In the case of the lever, the work done on the lever is called the *work input.* Work input is equal to the effort multiplied by the distance through which the lever is moved at the point where the effort is applied. For example, an applied effort of 10 pounds that moves the lever downward 1 foot gives 10 foot-pounds of work. This is true regardless of the length of mechanical advantage of the lever.

The work done by the lever is called the *work output.* The work output is equal to the resistance multiplied by the distance through

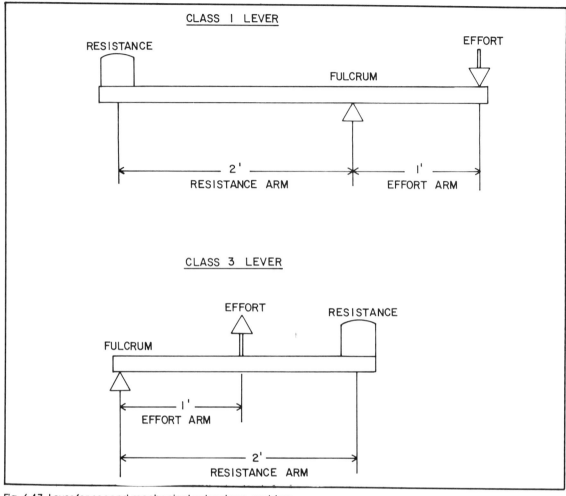

Fig. 6-17. Lever for second mechanical advantage problem.

which the resistance is moved. For example, a resistance of 10 pounds that is moved upward a distance of 1 foot gives 10 foot-pounds of work. This, also, is true regardless of the length or mechanical advantage of the lever.

The Wheel and Axle. The wheel and axle is a form of lever. The chainwheel on a bicycle, as shown in Fig. 6-18 is an example. The chain goes around the chainwheel. The radius of the chainwheel corresponds to the length of the resistance arm of a bar lever, as shown. The crank or pedal arm may be thought of as a point on an imaginary wheel. The crank or pedal arm measured from the center of the chainwheel to the pedal is the effort arm of a bar lever.

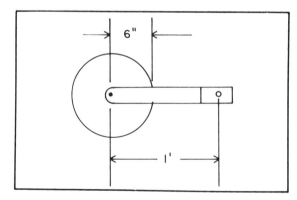

Fig. 6-18. Bicycle chainwheel is example of wheel and axle form of lever.

The mechanical advantage of this system, using the chainwheel as the axle and the pedal arm or crank as the wheel, can be calculated in exactly the same way as the mechanical advantage of a bar lever, which is the effort arm divided by the resistance arm. With the radius of the chainwheel 6 inches and the length of the crank pedal arm 1 foot, the mechanical advantage is 1 foot divided by 0.5 foot, which gives a mechanical advantage of 2.

Gears. Gears are wheels with teeth cut into the surface to prevent slipping. As is the case with the bar lever, gears can be used to increase force, to increase distance and/or speed, or to change the direction in which the force acts. An arrangement with a small gear with 12 teeth and a large gear with 24 teeth is shown in Fig. 6-19. When a force is applied to the small gear, the large gear gains force, but loses speed and distance.

With the same gear arrangement, when the force is applied to the large gear, the small gear gains speed and distance, but loses force.

In the above examples, the turning directions of the gear axles are reversed. Gears can also be arranged for perpendicular direction changes, as shown in Fig. 6-20.

The Pulley. A pulley is a wheel that is pivoted so that it is free to rotate about its center. Pulleys use the principle of the lever. Pulleys can be fixed to a permanent support or attached to a moving load. A fixed pulley can be compared to a Class One lever with the effort arm and resistance arm of the same length. A fixed pulley does not change the force; it only changes the direction of the force. The mechanical advantage is 1. Figure 6-21 shows a fixed pulley. Fixed

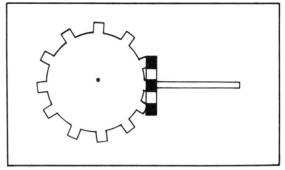

Fig. 6-20. Gears arranged for perpendicular direction change.

pulleys are often used in exercise machines and devices.

Movable pulleys can be arranged to give a mechanical advantage. An arrangement with one pulley is shown in Fig. 6-22. With a 10-pound resistance, a force of effort of 5 pounds (actually, slightly more is required to overcome the friction in the system—more on this later) is required to lift the resistance. When the effort is

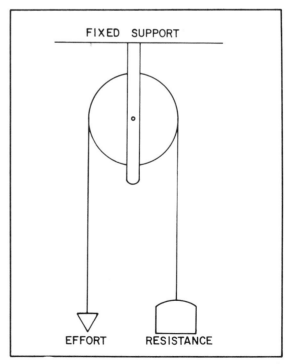

Fig. 6-21. Fixed pulley has mechanical advantage of one.

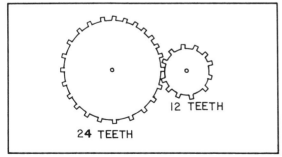

Fig. 6-19. Gear arrangement.

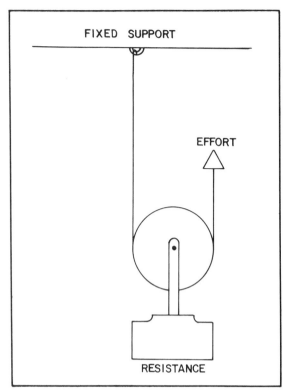

Fig. 6-22. Movable pulley arranged to give a mechanical advantage.

in Fig. 6-24. The mechanical advantage is equal to the number of ropes that support the resistance load.

INCLINED PLANES

Another class of simple machine is the *inclined plane*, which includes screws and wedges.

Inclined Plane. Figure 6-25 illustrates an inclined plane. Two dimensions are important—the height that the resistance load is lifted and the length of the inclined plane. For example, assume the load is lifted 5 feet. This is the resistance arm. The length of the inclined plane is 10 feet. This is the effort arm.

The effort is applied against a resistance, which in our example is 12 pounds. The resistance, in this case, is the force of gravity acting on the load.

The effort is the force that must be exerted to pull the load up the inclined plane, which in our example is 6 pounds. (Actually, a somewhat greater effort is required to overcome the friction in the system.)

moved upward 1 foot, however the resistance moves upward only 6 inches. This arrangement can be compared to a Class Two lever. There is a gain in force, but a loss of speed and distance. Notice that this is true regardless of the speed at which the effort is applied. The direction of the movement of the effort and resistance is the same.

Movable pulleys can be arranged to gain distance, as shown in Fig. 6-23. With a 5-pound resistance, a force of effort of 10 pounds is required to lift the resistance. When the effort is moved upward 6 inches, the resistance is moved upward 1 foot. This arrangement can be compared to a Class Three lever. There is a loss in force, but a gain in speed and distance. Notice that this is true regardless of the speed at which the effort is applied. The direction of the movement of the effort and the resistance is the same.

More than one pulley can be used in a system to gain mechanical advantage, as shown

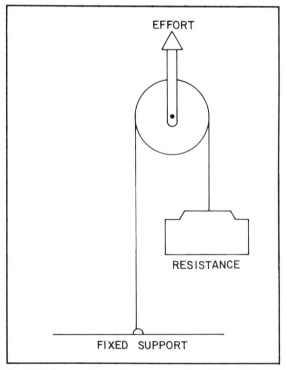

Fig. 6-23. A movable pulley arranged for giving distance.

130

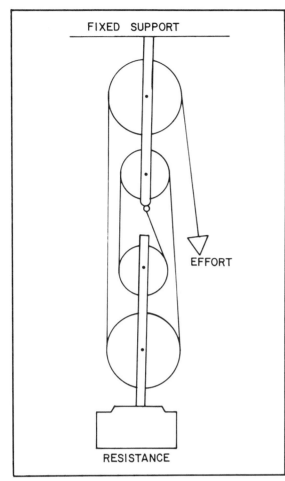

FIXED SUPPORT

EFFORT

RESISTANCE

Fig. 6-24. Pulleys arranged to give mechanical advantage of four.

The load or resistance is moved a distance of 10 feet along the inclined plane and at the same time it is raised a distance of 5 feet.

The mechanical advantage of the system is the effort arm divided by the resistance arm—in this example, 10 feet divided by 5 feet—which equals 2. The mechanical advantage is also equal to the resistance divided by the effort: 12 pounds divided by 6 pounds equals 2.

The work can also be calculated. The work input equals the force applied multiplied by the distance the force acted, which in our example is 6 pounds times 10 feet, equaling 60 foot-pounds.

The effort arm of the inclined plane is the actual distance through which the effort is applied, and the resistance arm is the actual distance through which the resistance is applied. Thus, the work input is equal to the effort moment, and the work output is equal to the resistance moment.

The Screw. A screw is an example of an inclined plane. The threads form an inclined plane wound around a cylinder. This can be compared to an inclined road that winds around a mountain. By means of a screw, a large resistance can be overcome by a small force.

As an example, we will use the type of jackscrew shown in Fig. 6-26. The *pitch* of the screw threads, the distance from one thread to the next, is 0.5 inch. With this pitch, one complete turn of the screw will lift the jackscrew 0.5 inch.

The jack handle is 16 inches long from the center of the jackscrew to the point where the effort is applied when turning the handle.

To determine how much load the jackscrew can lift, first calculate the mechanical advantage. You will first need to know the distance covered by the jack handle at the point where the effort is applied in one complete revolution. The handle is the effort arm and is equal to:

$$2 \times \pi \times r = 2 \times 3.14 \times 16 \text{ inches} = 100 \text{ inches.}$$

The effort arm is thus 100 inches long.

The distance that the jackscrew rises with one complete turn is the resistance arm, which in our example is 0.5 inch.

The mechanical advantage is the effort arm divided by the resistance arm—in our problem, 100 inches divided by 0.5 inches, which equals 200. The mechanical advantage is thus 200, which is a very large gain in force. If an effort of 5 pounds is applied to turn the jack handle, the load that the jackscrew can lift can be calculated using the law of levers—*resistance equals the effort arm multiplied by the effort divided by the resistance arm.* For our example the resistance equals 100 inches times 5 pounds divided by 0.5 inches, or 1,000 pounds.

From this, it can be seen that an effort of 5 pounds applied to the handle of the jack will raise a 1,000-pound load. For this gain in force, however, there is a very large loss in distance. The jack handle must be moved 200 inches to move the 1,000-pound load 1 inch.

The Wedge. Still another type of inclined plane is the wedge. A blade of an axe is a wedge— in reality, two inclined planes.

EFFICIENCY

To this point, we have assumed that the amount of useful work done by a machine (the output) is equal to the work input. In practice, however, the amount of useful work that we get out of a machine is always less than the amount of work put into it. The main problem is *friction*. Of course, in a well designed machine, this will be kept to a minimum to make the machine as efficient as possible.

Friction results from one surface rubbing against another surface. In the case of the bar lever, there is friction between the bar and the fulcrum; in axles, friction is caused by bearings. In each case, heat is generated. Part of the work, then, is converted into *heat energy*, which does not do useful work. To determine the useful work output, this lost energy must be subtracted from the work input.

The amount of friction depends on a number of variables that are difficult to account for. Losses due to friction can be kept to a minimum, however, by lubricating sliding surfaces, using bearings, and so on.

Energy loss can also result from moving the mass of the machine itself. For example, when bicycling up a hill, in addition to carrying the person pedaling,—the load—the weight of the machine, in this case the bicycle, must also be carried along. When a block and tackle that weighs 5 pounds is lifted 6 feet in order to lift a 200-pound load the same distance, 30-foot-pounds of work will be wasted in lifting the weight of the block and tackle.

The *efficiency* of a machine can be calculated by dividing the useful work output by the work input. To give a percentage, this number is then multiplied by 100. Thus, the *percent efficiency* equals the *useful work output divided by the work input times 100.* If the work input of a machine is 10-foot-pounds and the useful work output is 6-foot-pounds, the efficiency is $6/10 \times 100 = 60$ percent.

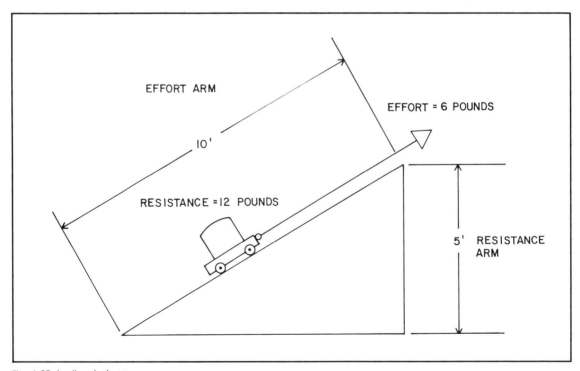

Fig. 6-25. Inclined plane.

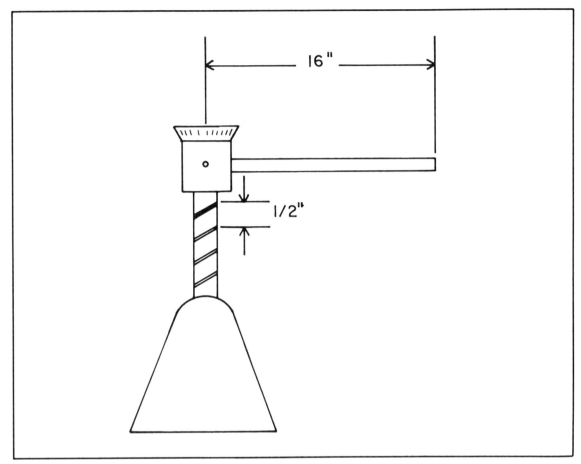

Fig. 6-26. A jackscrew that can be used to lift heavy loads.

This may seem very inefficient, but this would depend on the particular machine. Levers generally have a much higher efficiency, often approaching 100 percent, since there is very little friction at the fulcrum of many levers. It should be noted, however, that the efficiency will still always be less than 100 percent.

A jackscrew of the type described above and shown in Fig. 6-33 often has an efficiency of only about 40 to 50 percent. Even with this low efficiency, however, the jackscrew still results in a significant gain in force or mechanical advantage.

The following pieces of exercise equipment will apply the principles of the simple machines. By varying force, effort, and resistance these machines enable you to exercise specific muscles in very specific ways.

Chapter 7

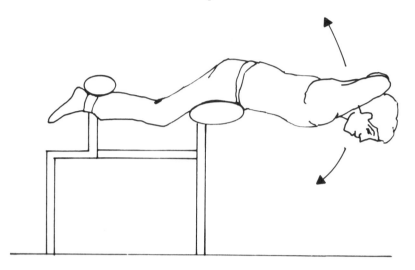

Weight and Pulley Machines

WEIGHT AND PULLEY DEVICES AND MACHINES ARE based on simple machines—the lever, pulley, wheel and axle, inclined plane and wedge, and screw. None of these machines have motors; *you* have to do the work—which is what exercise is all about. The machines and devices are used to monitor direction and resistance so that exercises can be more precisely controlled. Muscle groups can be isolated and exercised.

You may have seen motor driven treadmills and know that you can quickly drive anyone to exhaustion by using the appropriate grade and speed. But in this case, the motor is not doing the work for you. You must keep up with the speed of the turning belt, or end up off the back end. This is not the same thing as the passive resistance to a bicycle crank that is being turned by a motor at a certain speed. With your feet strapped to the pedals, they are pulled around by the motor. Unless you actively resist the turning, trying to stop it rather than let it carry your legs around, you are probably getting very little exercise.

The devices and machines detailed below do not have motors, so they do not share this problem. They are still machines, though. They allow us to gain (Fig. 7-1) or lose (Fig. 7-2) mechanical advantage with a corresponding loss or gain of speed and distance or move a resistance by applying the effort at various angles in relation to a resistance (Fig. 7-3). The resistance can be a weight (Fig. 7-4) moved against gravity, a spring or other elastic device (Fig. 7-5), or even your own body weight (Fig. 7-6). In some cases, the devices or machines are little more than "clamps" that hold your body in position to do a certain exercise, such as shown in Fig. 7-7.

WRIST ROLLER

A wrist roller device is shown in Fig. 7-8. The construction plan is shown in Fig. 7-9. The handle is a hardwood dowel 1½ inches in diameter and 14 inches long. A ⅜-inch diameter hole is drilled through the center of the dowel. A ⅜-inch diameter rope, about 5 feet long, is passed through the hole and double knotted so that it cannot slip back through. A clip is attached to the other end of the rope. This is passed through a weight plate and then clipped to the rope above the weight.

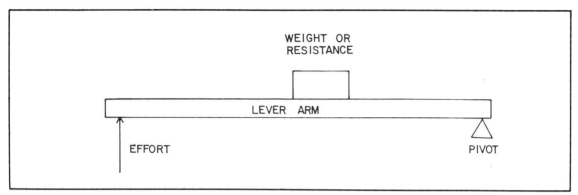

Fig. 7-1. Gain of mechanical advantage with corresponding loss of distance.

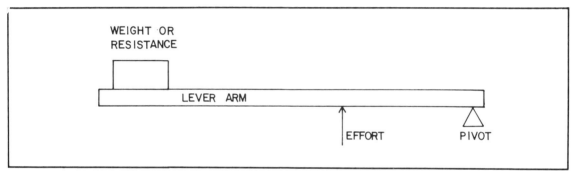

Fig. 7-2. Loss of mechanical advantage with corresponding gain of distance.

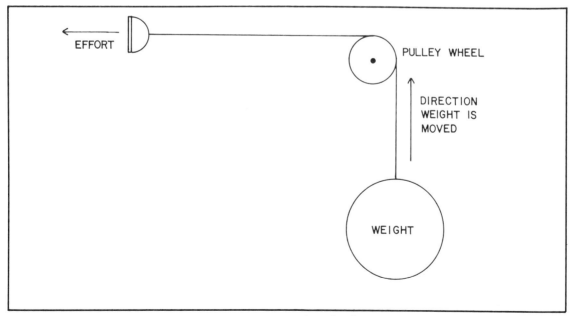

Fig. 7-3. Effort is applied in one direction to move weight another direction.

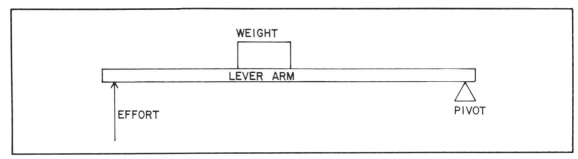

Fig. 7-4. Weight used as a resistance.

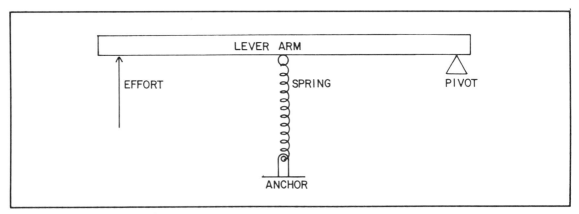

Fig. 7-5. Spring used as a resistance.

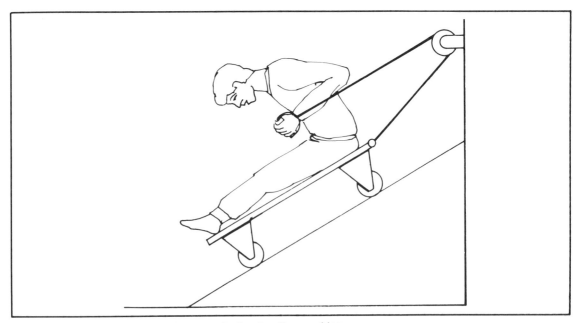

Fig. 7-6. Body weight used as resistance on inclined pulley machine.

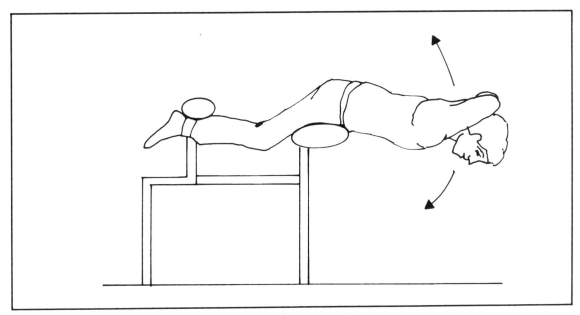

Fig. 7-7. Device for holding body in position for back extension exercise.

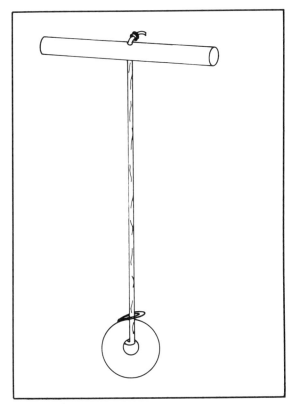

Fig. 7-8. Wrist roller exercise device.

The device is used for forearm and hand development. The basic exercise is to hold the bar in your hands as shown in Fig. 7-10 and roll the rope onto the handle to the point where the weight is at the handle. This device is based on the wheel and lever. The weight is raised straight up, yet the effort applied is a rolling motion of the wrists and hands.

KNEE EXTENSOR AND FLEXOR DEVICE

A knee extensor and flexor machine is shown in Fig. 7-11. The device can be connected to a flat padded weight training bench (see Chapter 4) or a specially constructed padded bench or table (Fig. 7-12). Figure 7-13 shows the device being used for knee extension exercise. Knee flexion exercise is shown in Fig. 7-14.

The arms are constructed from $1\frac{1}{2} \times \frac{1}{4}$-inch steel bar stock or from ¾-inch inside diameter steel pipe. The cross bars for the padded sections and weights are 1-inch outside diameter steel pipe or rod. The parts are cut and fitted and then brazed or welded together. Braces are used to reinforce the angles between the arms, as shown in Fig. 7-15. Holes are drilled to bolt the device to a bench or table so that it can pivot freely. The cross bars are wrapped with foam rubber, taped

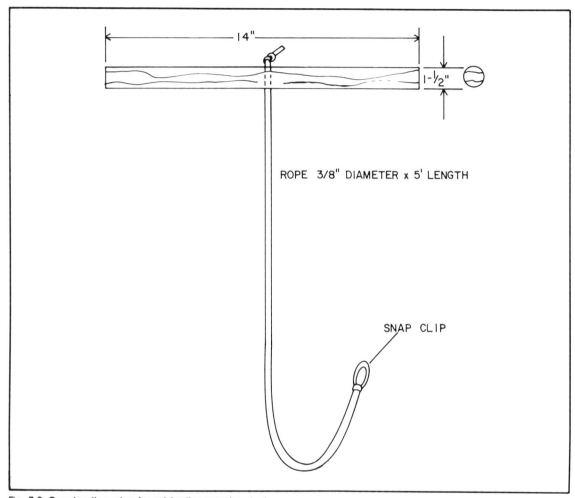

Fig. 7-9. Construction plan for wrist roller exercise device.

tightly in place (Fig. 7-16). Covers are then sewn from fabric backed vinyl or other suitable fabric.

Weight plates can be added to the ends of the weight bar and clamped in place with collars. When first doing knee flexor and extensor exercises, use only light weights. Gradually and progressively work up to heavier weights over a period of time.

LEVER BENCH PRESS MACHINE

Figure 7-17 shows a lever arm bench press machine. Using this machine gives you the safety advantage of not being able to drop the weight on yourself when doing bench presses,

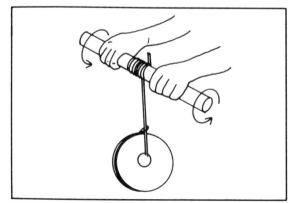

Fig. 7-10. Use of wrist roller.

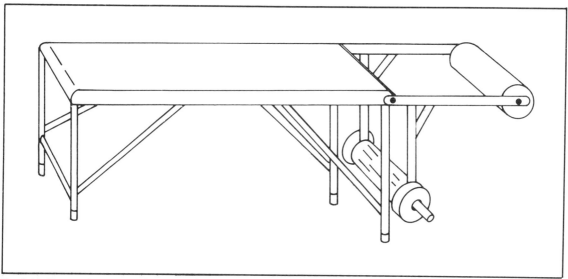

Fig. 7-11. Knee extensor and flexor machine.

because the stops limit the possible travel of the lifting handles. The basic frame for the machine is shown in Fig. 7-18. The joints are brazed or welded. The frame can be mounted to a floor (with floor flanges threaded on the ends of the pipe legs Fig. 7-19), to the floor and a wall (Fig. 7-20), or to a weight bench (Fig. 7-21). This is necessary so that the frame will not rise off the ground when bench presses are done.

The lever arm and lifting handles are shown in Fig. 7-22; the weight rack and attachment arm are detailed in Fig. 7-23. The rack allows you to add or subtract weight plates, as desired. Notice that because the weight rack is attached to the lever arm between the pivot point and the handles where the lifting effort is applied, the weight lifted will be less than the weight placed on the platform. A guide for the weight rack and

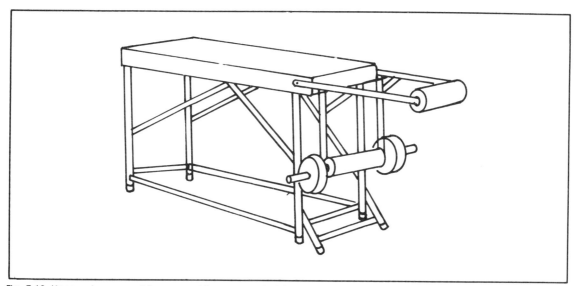

Fig. 7-12. Knee extensor and flexor machine connected to specially constructed table.

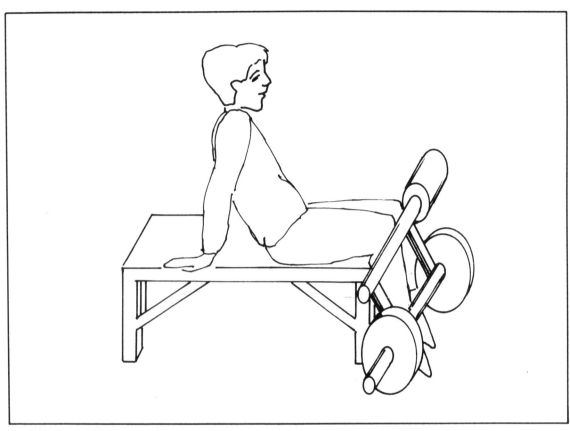

Fig. 7-13. Knee extension exercise.

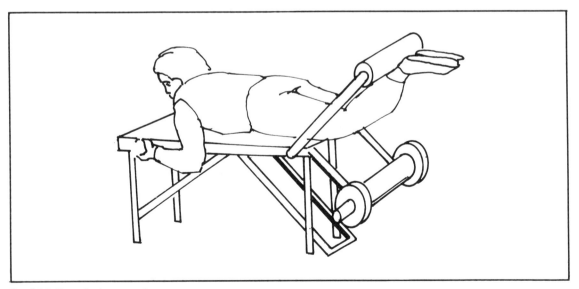

Fig. 7-14. Knee flexion exercise.

140

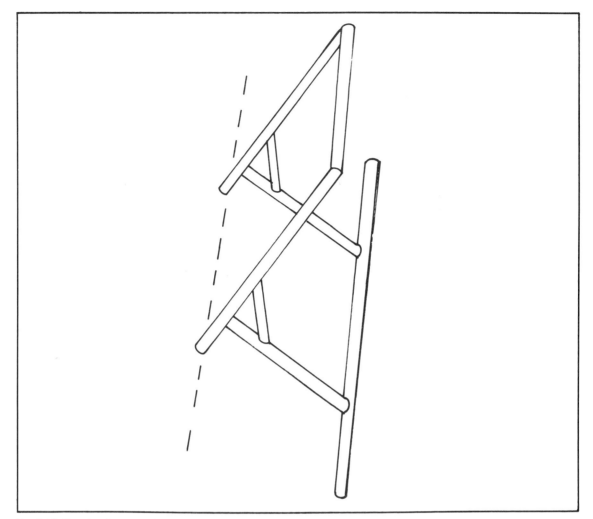

Fig. 7-15. Construction plan for arms and mounting bars.

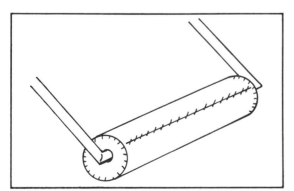

Fig. 7-16. Cross bar is wrapped with foam rubber and a cover is used.

arm is detailed in Fig. 7-24. This is adjusted by means of bolts that pass through holes (Fig. 7-25). Additional safety or limiting stops can also be used on the frame, as shown in Fig. 7-26. These can also be made adjustable (Fig. 7-27). Bicycle handlebar grips are used on the lifting handles (Fig. 7-28). The grips should be glued to the bars so that they cannot turn or slip off.

LEVER SQUAT MACHINE

Figure 7-29 shows a lever squat machine. This arrangement offers the advantage over using a regular barbell in that you cannot drop the weight with the machine.

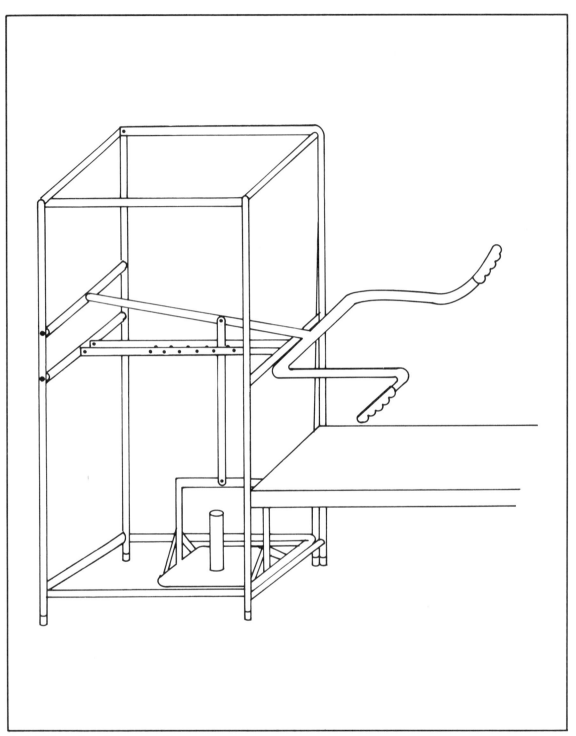

Fig. 7-17. Lever bench press machine.

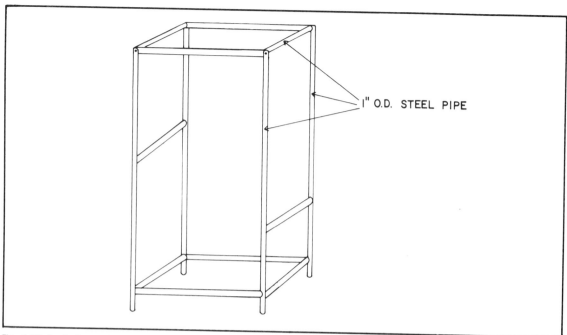

Fig. 7-18. Basic frame for lever bench press machine.

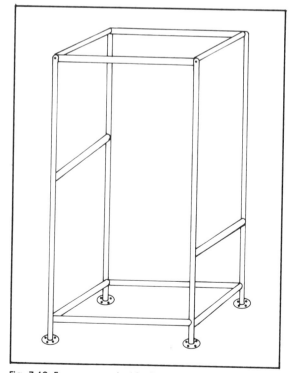

Fig. 7-19. Frame mounted to floor with pipe flanges.

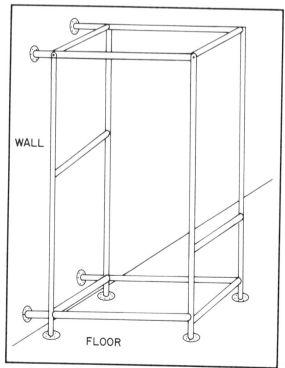

Fig. 7-20. Frame mounted to floor and wall.

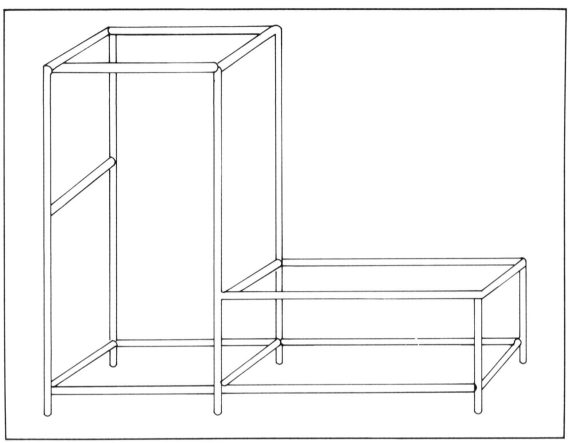

Fig. 7-21. Frame mounted to bench.

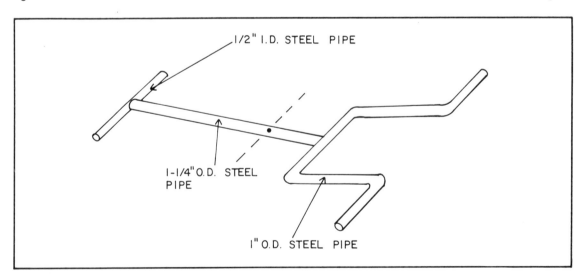

1/2" I.D. STEEL PIPE

1-1/4" O.D. STEEL PIPE

1" O.D. STEEL PIPE

Fig. 7-22. Lever arm and lifting handle.

144

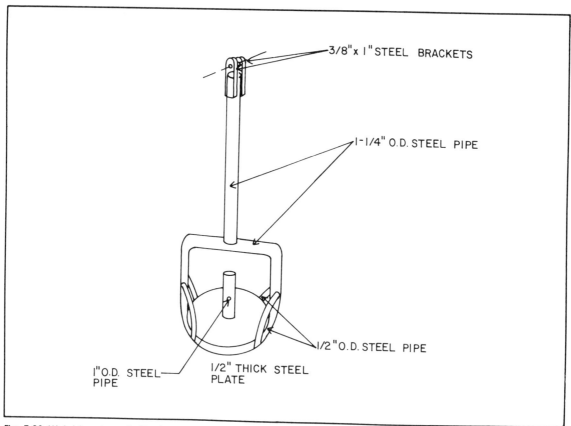

Fig. 7-23. Weight rack and attachment arm.

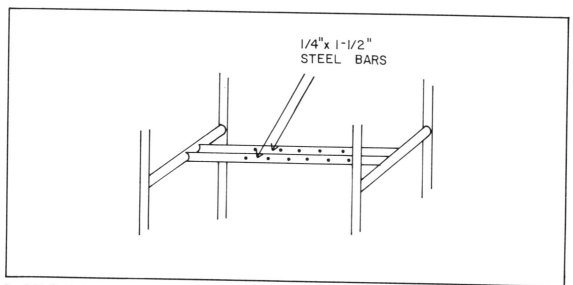

Fig. 7-24. Guide for weight arm.

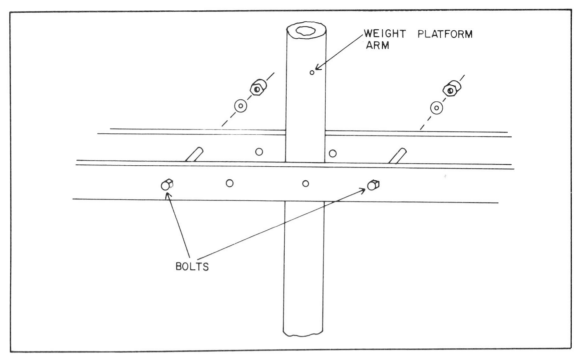

Fig. 7-25. Stop adjustment bolts in arm guide.

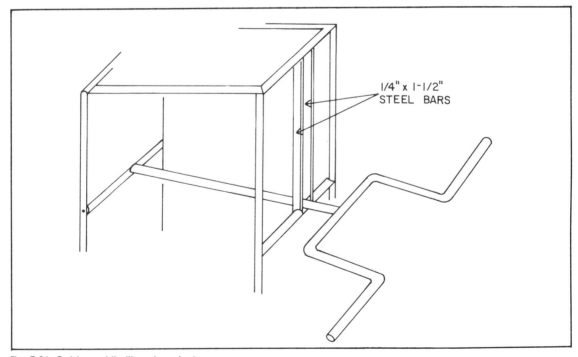

Fig. 7-26. Guide and limiting stops for lever.

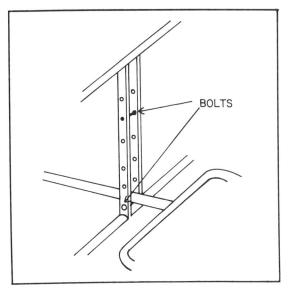

Fig. 7-27. Stop adjustment bolts used on lever guide.

The basic frame for the lever squat machine is shown in Fig. 7-30. The frame is assembled by brazing or welding. The frame must be firmly mounted: a floor mounting with floor flanges threaded on the ends of the pipe frame posts and bolted or screwed to the floor is shown in Fig. 7-31. A floor and wall mounting is shown in Fig. 7-32. A solid mounting is necessary to keep the frame from lifting off the floor when the weight is lifted.

The lever arm and lifting frame and handles are shown in Fig. 7-33. The lever arm is attached to the frame so that it can pivot. The lifting frame is padded with foam rubber for the shoulders (Fig. 7-34). This should be taped in place, then covered with fabric backed plastic vinyl or other suitable covering material. Bicycle handlebar grips are installed on the handles (Fig. 7-35).

The weight arm and weight platform construction is shown in Fig. 7-36. This is attached to the lever arm so that it can pivot. A guide and adjustable stop for the weight arm is shown in Fig. 7-37. The weight platform allows you to add and subtract weight plates, as desired. Because of the placement of the weight arm on the lever arm, the amount of weight lifted (effort applied at the shoulder rack and hand grips) will be less than that used on the weight platform.

An adjustable limit stop for the lever arms is used to adjust the lower limit to which the lever arms can go, as shown in Fig. 7-38. This stop is adjusted for the bottom limit you wish to reach during the squat exercise. This can be half-squats, three-quarter squats, or full squats, as desired.

The construction detailed above will handle moderate amounts of weight. For squat exercises with heavy weights of 150 pounds or over, the construction should be beefed up with larger diameter and stronger steel pipe and heavier materials.

The machine can also be modified for standing press exercises, curls, and other exercises that are typically done with barbells.

PULLEY MACHINES

Pulley machines are useful exercise equipment. As a general rule, these change the direction the resistance is moved in relation to the applied effort. The weights are usually moved straight up against the force of gravity. It is very desirable in certain exercises to be able to apply the effort at a different angle.

A basic downward pull pulley machine (Fig. 7-39) is often called a *latissimus dorsi machine* because of the muscles that are exercised by pulling downward. It does not change

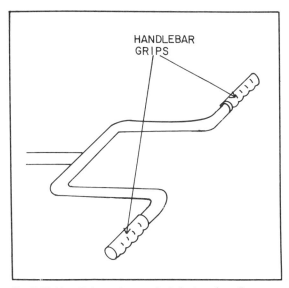

Fig. 7-28. Handlebar grips are installed on handles.

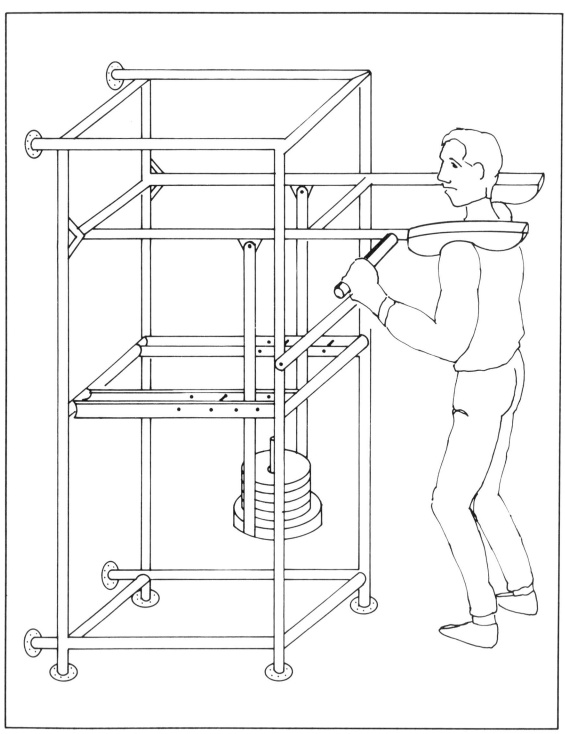

Fig. 7-29. Lever squat machine.

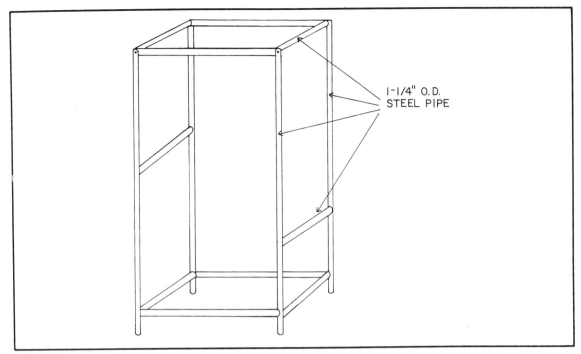

Fig. 7-30. Basic frame for lever squat machine.

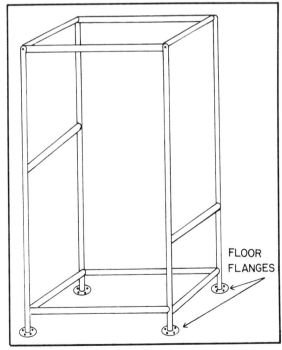

Fig. 7-31. Floor mounting of frame.

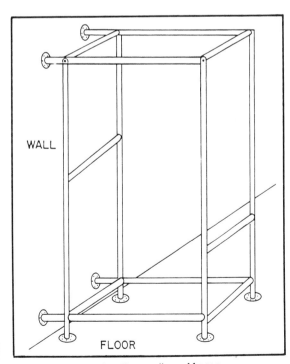

Fig. 7-32. Floor and wall mounting of frame.

149

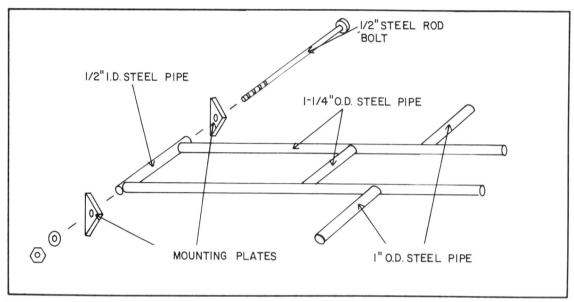

Fig. 7-33. Lever arms and lifting frame.

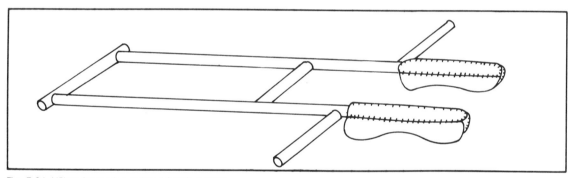

Fig. 7-34. Lifting frame is padded for shoulders.

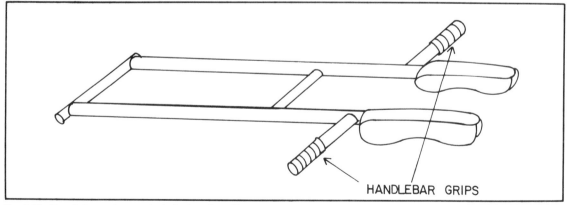

Fig. 7-35. Handlebar grips are installed on handles.

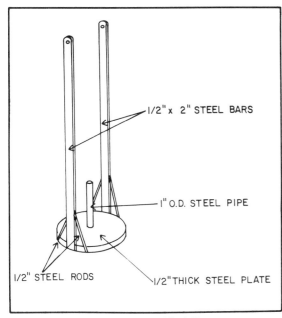

Fig. 7-36. Weight arms and weight platform.

the mechanical advantage. The machine could be constructed with one pulley, but this does not get the weight out of the way of the person doing the exercise.

The two heavy-duty pulleys are securely attached to a ceiling beam or specially constructed mounting frame, which in turn is securely attached to the floor, wall, or ceiling. The pulleys should be some distance apart so that the weight cannot fall on the person doing the exercise.

Either regular polyester rope can be used, or you can use flexible wire rope. Wire rope is recommended if heavy weights are to be used. Some pulleys are designed for regular rope and others for wire rope, and for specific sizes. Make certain that you select pulleys that will work with the rope or wire rope that you intend to use. For a typical exercise machine with light and moderately heavy weights, ⅜-inch diameter polyester rope designed for running sailboat

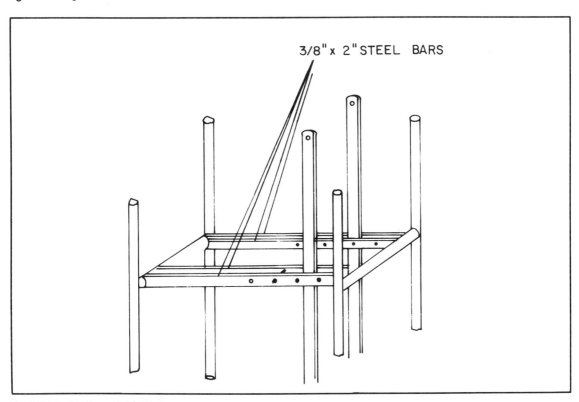

Fig. 7-37. Guide for weight arms.

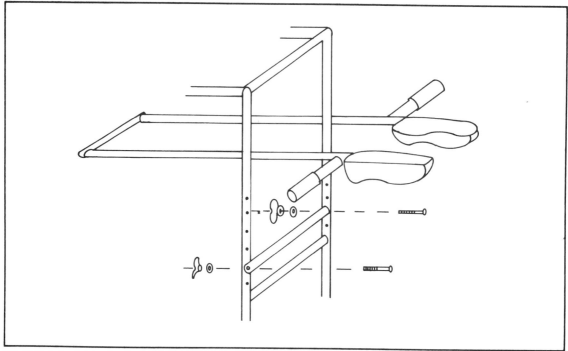

Fig. 7-38. Adjustable stop for lever arms.

rigging, or 3/16-inch flexible steel aircraft cable (7 × 19 arrangement), are about right. Regular rope, wire rope, pulleys, clamps, and fittings can be purchased from marine and hardware stores.

The handle for the single rope or cable pulley machine is 1¼-inch outside diameter steel pipe with a closed-ring eye bolt installed through a hole in the center of the pipe, as shown in Fig. 7-40. Rope is attached to this by means of a knot or splice. A rope thimble is used over the eye to protect the rope (Fig. 7-41). For cable, cable clamps (Fig. 7-42) or swagging fittings are attached with special swagging tools or presses.

The weight platform is a pipe flange and section of 1-inch outside diameter steel pipe, as shown in Fig. 7-43. A wooden base is attached to the floor flange with through bolts, as shown in Fig. 7-44. The bottom of the wood is padded with heavy foam rubber and covered with heavy canvas material (Fig. 7-45). This will help to prevent breakage if the weight is accidentally dropped. A steel ring is welded to the upper end of the weight pipe for attachment of the rope or

cable (Fig. 7-46). A heavy-duty hook or clasp is attached to the weight end of the rope or cable for quick and easy removal of weight plates. The weight platform is often caged, as shown in Fig. 7-47, so that there is no danger of the weights dropping on the person exercising or anyone else in the area.

As a general rule, use less weight than your body weight. If you use more weight than your body weight, the machine will pull you off the ground unless you are supported in some manner. Figures 7-48 and 7-49 show typical exercises with the single cable pulley machine.

Similar machines can be constructed using two parallel pulley systems with individual handles, as shown in Fig. 7-50. Construction is similar to that of the single rope or cable system detailed above. Additional pulleys can be added without changing the mechanical advantage to allow exercising with different pulling angles, such as shown in Figs. 7-51 and 7-52. The construction plan for making the handles from wood is shown in Fig. 7-53, and from metal, in Fig. 7-54.

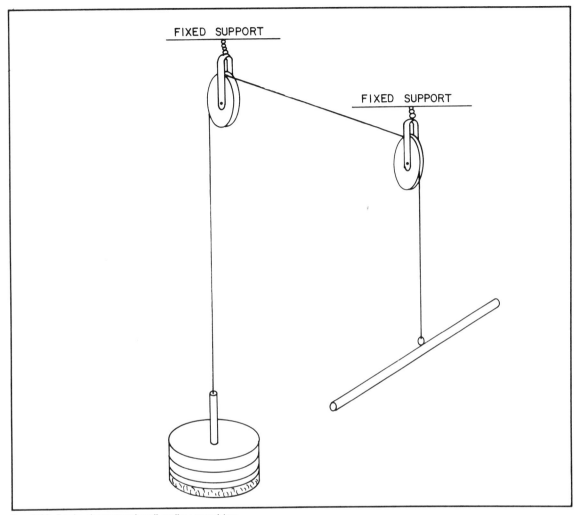

Fig. 7-39. Basic downward pull pulley machine.

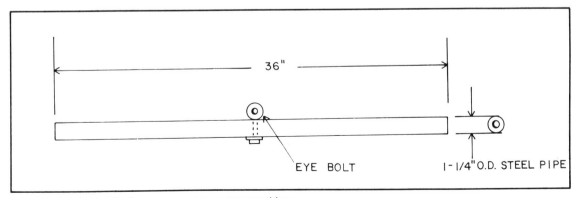

Fig. 7-40. Handle for single rope or cable pulley machine.

153

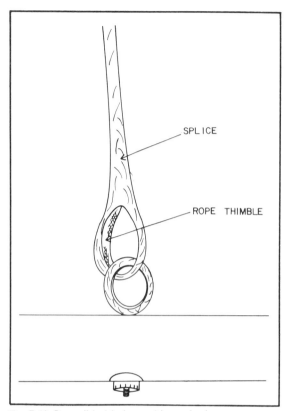

Fig. 7-41. Rope thimble is used to protect rope.

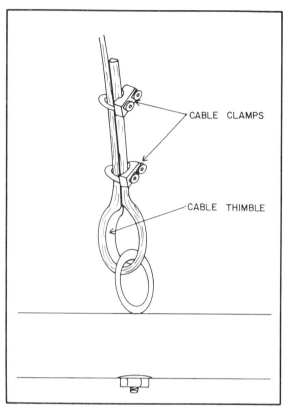

Fig. 7-42. Wire rope connected by cable clamps.

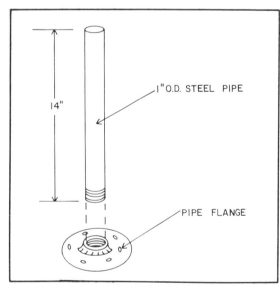

Fig. 7-43. Weight platform for pulley machine.

A pulley machine for leg extension exercises is shown in Fig. 7-55. While this uses four pulleys for the single cable, the mechanical advantage is still 1. The bench must be firmly mounted either to the floor or to a frame that has the weight pulleys attached.

A somewhat different pulley machine consists of an inclined board with a movable seat, as shown in Fig. 7-56. In this case, your body weight is used as the resistance. Since the inclined board gives you a mechanical advantage, you will be pulling considerably less than your actual body weight. The resistance can be changed by changing the angle of incline.

Construction of the inclined board is similar to that of the adjustable sit-up platform detailed in Chapter 4, except that the board is not padded and a guide rail of 1 × 2-inch hardwood is added to the center of the board, as shown in Fig. 7-57.

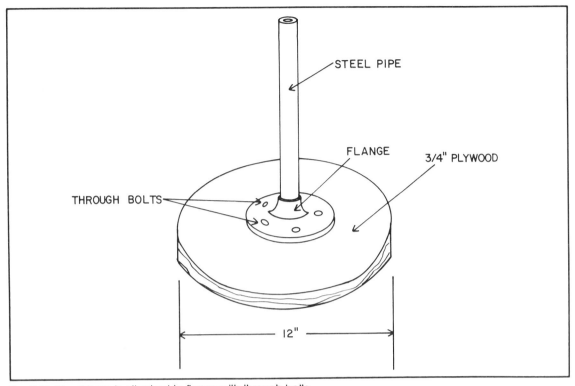

Fig. 7-44. Wood base is attached to flange with through bolts.

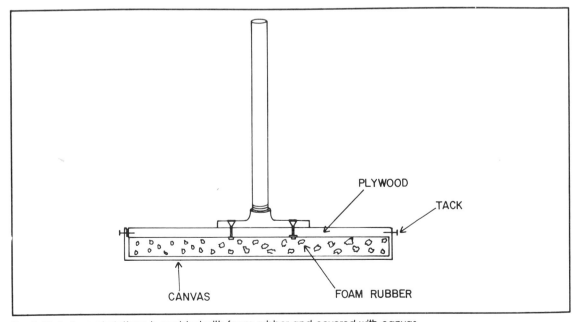

Fig. 7-45. Bottom of platform is padded with foam rubber and covered with canvas.

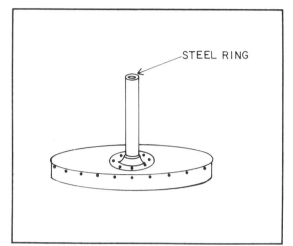

Fig. 7-46. Steel ring is welded to top of weight pipe.

Fig. 7-47. Front half of weight rack is caged.

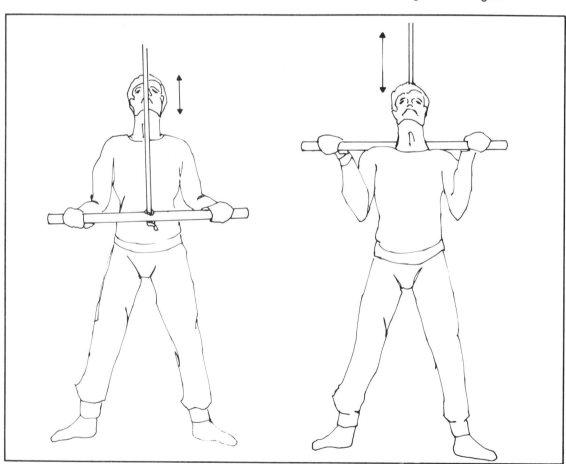

Fig. 7-48. In front of body exercise on pulley weight machine and behind head exercise on pulley weight machine.

156

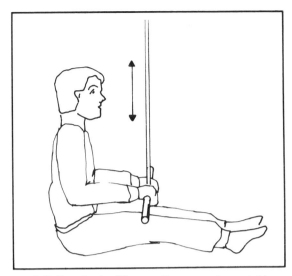

Fig. 7-49. Exercise in sitting position on pulley weight machine.

The construction plan for the movable board is shown in Fig. 7-58. This has two rail guides that fit over the rail on the slant board. Non-turning caster wheels are attached to the movable board. The seat is padded (Fig. 7-59). Eye bolts are attached to the movable board for attaching the ropes (Fig. 7-60). The pulleys attach to eye bolts in the upper end of the slant board, as shown in Fig. 7-61. Individual handles, as detailed above for parallel pulley machines, are attached to the ends of the ropes.

A typical exercise using the slant board with movable platform is shown in Fig. 7-62. By reversing your direction, a pulling or rowing motion can be done (Fig. 7-63).

TREADMILL

A treadmill is included here only to present a complete line of built-it-yourself exercise equip-

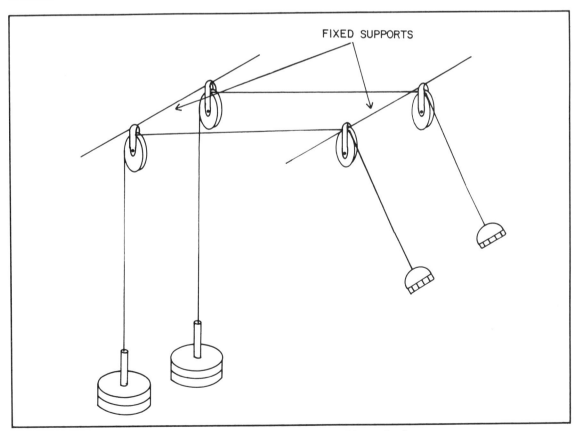

FIXED SUPPORTS

Fig. 7-50. Machine with two sets of pulleys and ropes running parallel to each other.

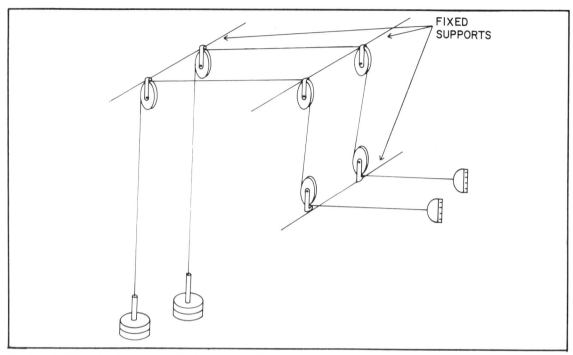

Fig. 7-51. Additional pulleys added for horizontal pulling.

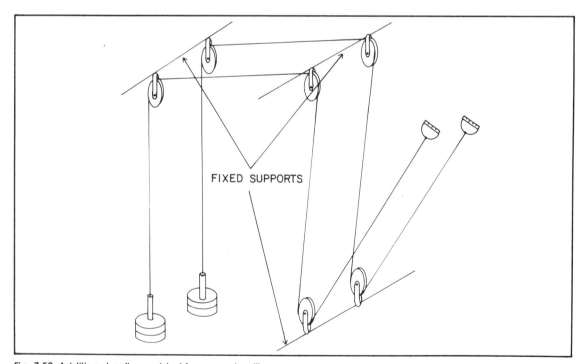

Fig. 7-52. Additional pulleys added for upward pulling.

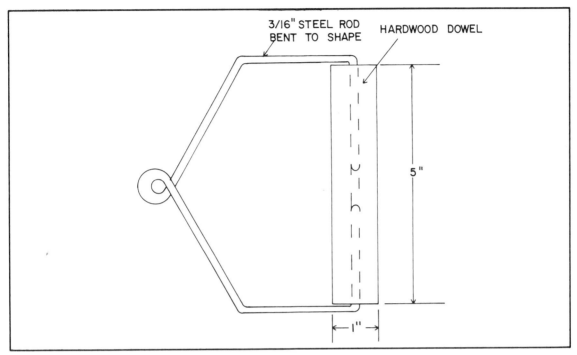

Fig. 7-53. Handle constructed for pulley machine.

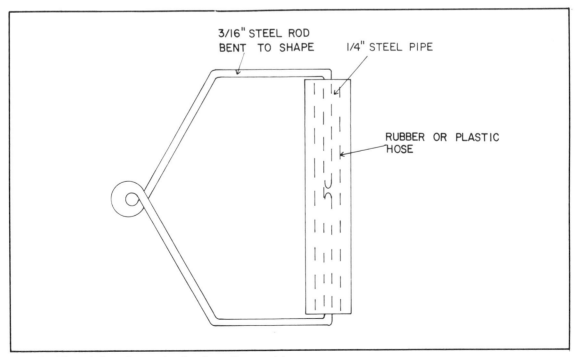

Fig. 7-54. Alternate handle construction for pulley machine.

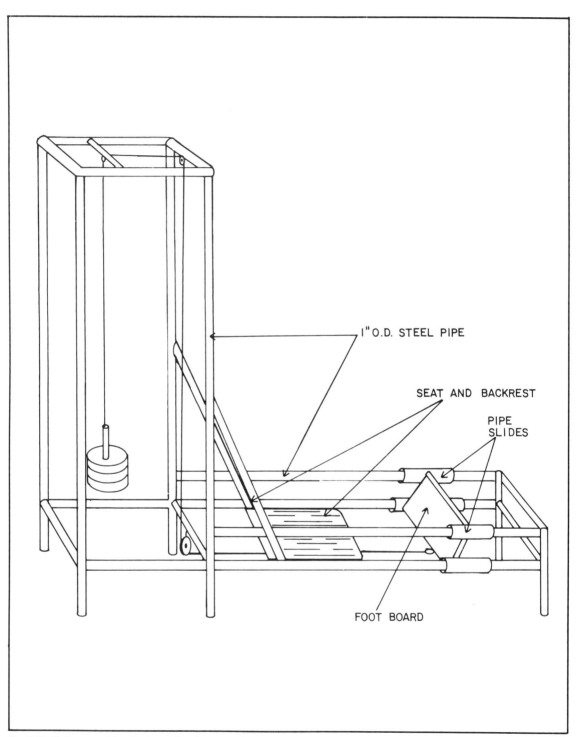

1" O.D. STEEL PIPE

SEAT AND BACKREST

PIPE SLIDES

FOOT BOARD

Fig. 7-55. Pulley machine for leg extension exercise.

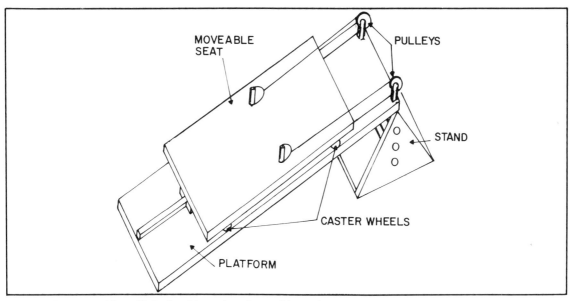

Fig. 7-56. Pulley machine with inclined board and movable seat.

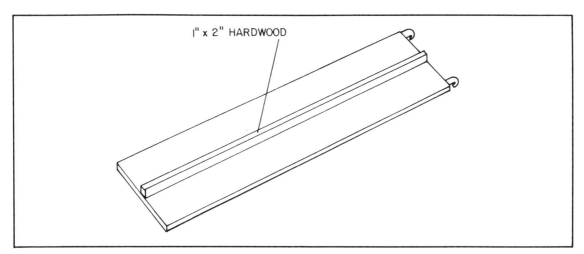

Fig. 7-57. Guide board is used on platform.

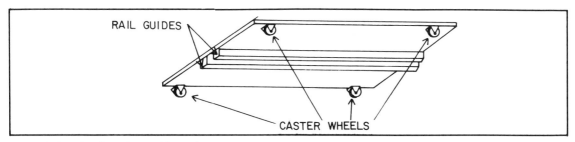

Fig. 7-58. Construction of movable seat.

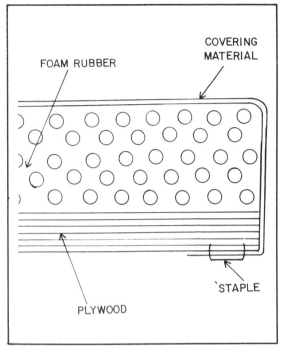

Fig. 7-59. The seat is padded and covered with plastic material.

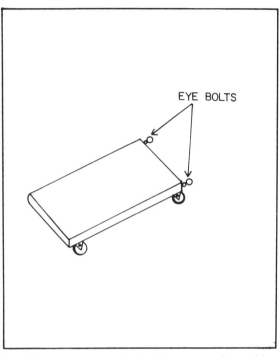

Fig. 7-60. Eye bolts are attached to corners of movable seat.

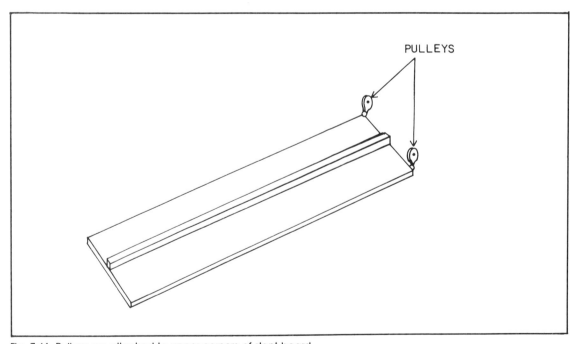

Fig. 7-61. Pulleys are attached to upper corners of slant board.

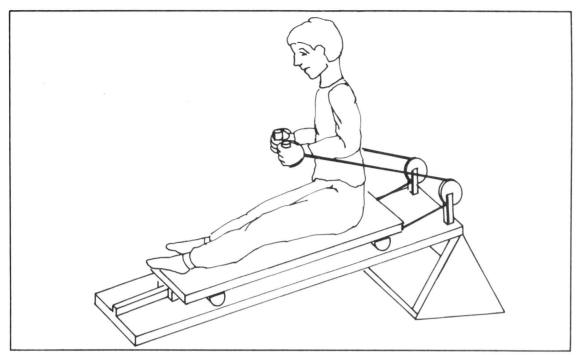

Fig. 7-62. Exercise facing downward on slant board.

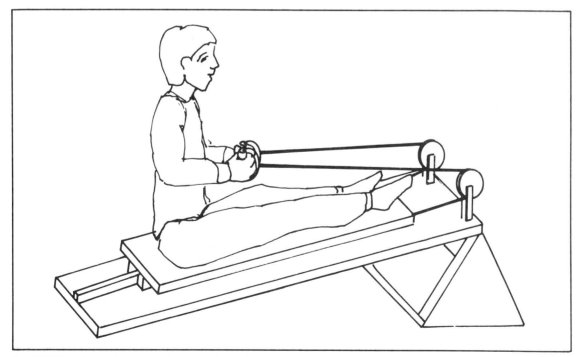

Fig. 7-63. Exercise facing upward on slant board.

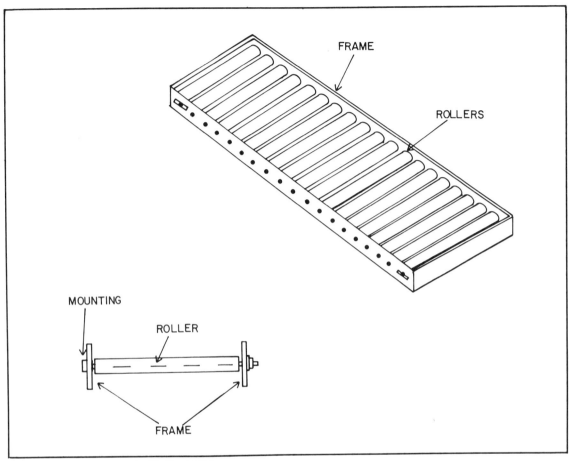

Fig. 7-64. Rollers are mounted to the frame.

ment. A treadmill is quite difficult to construct and, in my opinion, offers almost no advantages over just plan walking and jogging.

The treadmill consists of a series of rollers that are mounted to a frame so that the rollers can turn freely. The rollers at one or both ends should be adjustable so that the belt can be tightened. The mounting frame can be wood or metal, as desired. The construction is shown in Fig. 7-64.

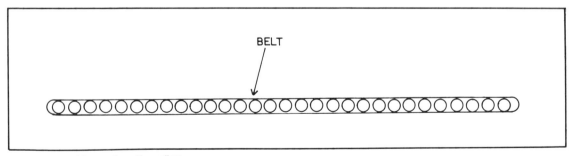

Fig. 7-65. A belt is used on the rollers.

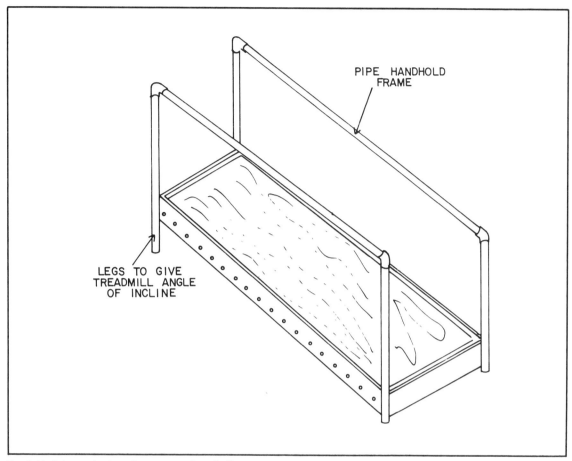

PIPE HANDHOLD
FRAME

LEGS TO GIVE
TREADMILL ANGLE
OF INCLINE

Fig. 7-66. A frame for handholds on a treadmill.

A wide conveyor-type belt is used over the rollers, as shown in Fig. 7-65. The tension should be adjusted so that the belt will turn freely, yet give a firm walking surface.

A handhold pipe frame is added to the treadmill, as shown in Fig. 7-66. The forward legs are often used to give the treadmill an inclined angle, as shown.

165

Chapter 8

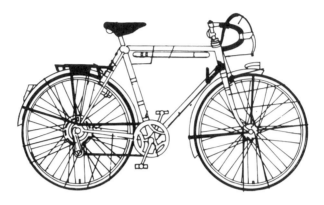

Bicycles

A BICYCLE PROVIDES IDEAL CARDIOVASCULAR AND endurance exercise. To receive the maximum benefit from cycling, you will need a place where you can bicycle at moderate or high speeds for long periods of time. For this type of bicycling, you will probably want to have a bicycle that is as efficient as possible. For anything less than ideal riding conditions, you may want to consider a bicycle that is less efficient (equivalent to using more resistance on a stationary exercise pedal cycle). A bicycle with changeable gear ratios, such as a 10-speed, can offer the best of both worlds. When you have a place safe for long-distance high-speed riding, you can use the gears that give the greatest efficiency. When you have conditions that do not allow high-speed riding, you can deliberately use a wrong gear to make the riding more difficult, that is, with a greater workload.

THE BEST BICYCLE FOR YOU

The first problem is finding the right bicycle for your budget and your needs. This depends on how you intend to use the bicycle and how much

you can afford to spend. It's possible to have too much bicycle for your intended use, as well as too little. For ordinary exercise and physical fitness riding, an expensive touring machine is probably more bicycle than you need, at least when you are first starting out. The lighter weight and greater precision make it more delicate, and it requires more care and maintenance than a heavier, less precise machine. A delicate machine also leads to greater problems in protecting it from wear, damage from the environment, and theft.

Performance is a combination of rider and bicycle. Important factors for the bicycle include design, precision, quality of construction, weight, and condition. The bicycle can be considered an extension of the rider's most powerful muscles. The combination of the rider and the bicycle is very effective for transferring the linear motion machine—the human body—into the rotary motion of the bicycle wheels. The human body, of course, is far more versatile when not on a bicycle and is capable of many diverse actions, such as walking, running, or climbing stairs and ladders. A bicycle is far more limited and must always be combined with a person to generate a source of power. On smooth hard surfaces that are level or of limited grade, however, a bicycle can transfer human power input into very effective and efficient motion.

Bicycles are a series of compromises. A person who wants a bicycle for exercise or physical fitness is faced with a seemingly endless number of choices. To complicate the matter, there is no simple way to classify bicycles. To sort out the picture, I will first discuss bicycles in a general way before going on to the specifics of design and construction.

Single-Speed Bicycles

Single-speed bicycles (Fig. 8-1) have long been popular. This bicycle has only one fixed gear ratio. (Gear ratios are explained later in this chapter.)

There was a time when most single-speed bicycles had *balloon tires* and were called "heavyweights" or "American" bicycles. Today, single-speed bicycles are more likely to be middleweights, and there are even some lightweight models on the market. Light weight is an advantage in bicycle performance.

A single-speed bicycle of the same shape, weight, and precision will have the same performance as a multi-geared bicycle ridden in the same gear ratio. This might seem obvious, but it is a fact often overlooked. Many people believe that a 10-speed bicycle, disregarding the ability to change gear ratios, is automatically a better performing bicycle. This is because, if we disregard single-speed track racing bicycles, few medium-priced and almost no high-priced bi-

cycles are available in single-speed models. The reverse, however, is not true: many low-priced bicycles feature gearing systems.

Single-speed bicycles generally have coaster brakes that work by back pedaling. This is an extremely convenient arrangement that allows both pedaling and braking by foot action. These bicycles can often be identified by the absence of hand-operated brake levers, although some coaster brakes are supplemented with a *caliper brake* on the front wheel with one hand-lever control on the handlebars. Many coaster brakes have an arm extension from the rear hub that connects to the bicycle frame.

Another type of single-speed bicycle is the *fixed sprocket* (non-freewheeling) track racing cycle. These fixed hubs are generally found only on bicycles designed for this special purpose and should not be confused with freewheeling single-speed bicycles. Freewheeling allows the wheel to continue turning even when you aren't pedaling. This coasting is a tremendous advantage for normal riding.

The main advantages of single-speed bikes when compared to bicycles with changeable gear ratios is that they have no complicated gear changing mechanisms and, on most models, brake by simple back pedaling. The main disadvantage is that all riding must be done in a single gear ratio.

For many purposes, especially for limited exercise riding on fairly level surfaces, the single-speed is all that is needed. For longer rides, higher speeds, and climbing hills, however, the advantages of being able to change gear ratios will quickly become apparent.

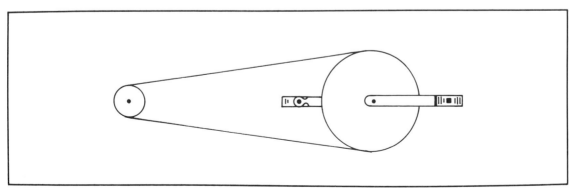

Fig. 8-1. Single-speed bicycle has only one gear ratio.

Internal Hub Multi-Speed Bicycles

The next improvement—or complication, depending on how you look at it—is *internal hub gearing*. This gearing most commonly offers three speeds or gear ratios. It is also available with two-gear and five-gear ratios. Most of these are shifted by finger levers. Models that shift automatically have been introduced from time to time, but these have never proven popular and/or satisfactory.

Internal hub multi-speed gears generally present more difficult adjustment, maintenance, and repair problems than single speeds, but they offer the advantage of a choice of gear ratios.

Bikes with internal hub gearing are ideal when something more than a single gear ratio is needed, but something less than a 10-speed is adequate. While internal hub gears make riding slightly more complicated than single-speed bicycles, they are generally much easier to operate than are *derailleur systems* (detailed later in this chapter).

A few years back, internally geared bikes were representative of a type of bicycle called the *English racer*. Today, however, internal gears are used on many different styles of bicycles, and they are no longer representative of a specific type of bicycle. As is the case with single-speeds (other than fixed-hub track bicycles), the internal hub geared bicycles are generally only available in the lower price and lower quality ranges. They often extend a notch or two above what is available in single-speeds, however, with correspondingly higher price tags.

In general, the advantages of internal hub gears over derailleur systems are ease of adjustment and operation. Disadvantages are a smaller number of gear choices and difficulty in making internal repairs when they break down—which fortunately isn't often.

Derailleur Bicycles

The next general type, and presently the most popular, is the 10-speed with derailleur gears. While other numbers of gears—especially five and fifteen—are also used, the 10-speed has become the general standard. The rear *derailleur* (the shift mechanism at the rear sprocket) generally has five sprockets. The front derailleur has

two, resulting in a total of 10 possible gear combinations. With a single chainwheel at the crank and the same five sprockets at the rear hub, the set up becomes a 5-speed. The same set up with three chainwheels at the crank becomes a 15-speed. While the five cluster rear sprocket arrangement is the most common, other numbers are sometimes used.

Derailleur systems are generally both more difficult to operate and keep in adjustment than internal hub gears. Derailleur systems are often easier to repair than internal hub gears, though. Many of the newer designs of derailleurs, even on inexpensive bikes, have been greatly improved over earlier versions. Some of the better designs approach the ease of operation of hub gears.

I recommend 10-speed bicycles for general exercise and physical fitness riding for those who are reasonably fit and agile, and especially for those who intend to ride long distances, at high speeds, or on rolling or hilly terrain.

Riding Posture

In selecting a bicycle, the riding posture you intend to use is an important consideration. "Pure" bicyclists are fond of pointing out that there is only one type of saddle (narrow) and position (high) that is proper for bicycling. This is probably true from an efficiency point of view, but it's not necessarily the most comfortable. Many riders have neither the desire nor the necessary fitness to ride like this.

Some bicycles are designed to be ridden in a fairly erect position. These generally have wide, (Fig. 8-2) fairly low saddles and flat or slightly upturned handlebars (Fig. 8-3). These bicycles are sometimes considered beginners' bicycles, but I think they have important uses beyond this. I know of a number of older adults, for example, who do bicycling for exercise and physical fitness on a regular basis who are incapable of the so-called "racing" posture.

The second main category of bicycles you will want to consider for exercise and physical fitness riding have narrow *touring* or *racing saddles* and dropped (down-turned) handlebars. This arrangement actually offers a variety of riding positions, from fairly upright to leaning

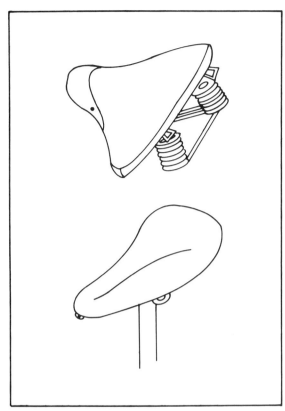

Fig. 8-2. Wide saddle and narrow saddle.

far forward. This saddle and handlebar combination is recommended for those who have the necessary fitness and agility to use it.

Wide saddles are seldom used with dropped handlebars; the arrangement isn't very practical. Narrow saddles are sometimes used advantageously with flat or slightly upturned handlebars, though.

Intended Use

Bicycles are designed and constructed for specific uses. Some bicycles, for example, are intended for short rides and utility use. Others are designed specifically for touring or racing. There are subtle and not so subtle differences in each category. While most designs will serve for exercise and physical fitness riding, some are more suitable than others. I recommend touring designs for those just starting out in exercise and physical fitness riding.

Price and Quality

As a general rule, a higher priced bicycle will be of higher quality. There are some exceptions to this, however, especially in the lower price brackets. While these figures are somewhat arbitrary, it may be helpful to consider bicycles that cost under $150 as being low-priced, $150 to $250 as being medium-priced, and over $250 as being high-priced. These price ranges roughly parallel distinct quality categories of bicycles.

COMPARISON

So far, you should have a general idea of the differences in bicycles. I suggest that you study these points and then apply them when shopping at bicycle shops, bicycle shows, and elsewhere. Before you actually select a bicycle to buy, however, it's important to go one long step further and be able to judge and compare the frame and components that make up a specific bicycle.

Frames

The *frame*, which for our purposes here will also include the front fork, is the basic part or

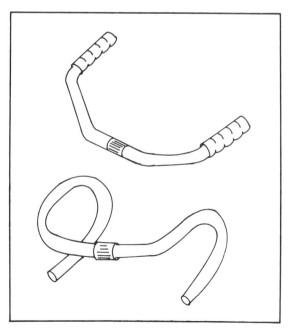

Fig. 8-3. Slightly upturned handlebars, and dropped or down-turned handlebars.

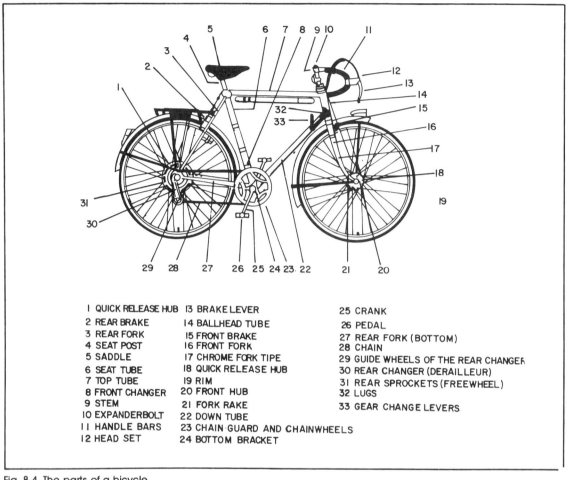

Fig. 8-4. The parts of a bicycle.

1 QUICK RELEASE HUB	13 BRAKE LEVER	25 CRANK
2 REAR BRAKE	14 BALLHEAD TUBE	26 PEDAL
3 REAR FORK	15 FRONT BRAKE	27 REAR FORK (BOTTOM)
4 SEAT POST	16 FRONT FORK	28 CHAIN
5 SADDLE	17 CHROME FORK TIPE	29 GUIDE WHEELS OF THE REAR CHANGER
6 SEAT TUBE	18 QUICK RELEASE HUB	30 REAR CHANGER (DERAILLEUR)
7 TOP TUBE	19 RIM	31 REAR SPROCKETS (FREEWHEEL)
8 FRONT CHANGER	20 FRONT HUB	32 LUGS
9 STEM	21 FORK RAKE	33 GEAR CHANGE LEVERS
10 EXPANDERBOLT	22 DOWN TUBE	
11 HANDLE BARS	23 CHAIN GUARD AND CHAINWHEELS	
12 HEAD SET	24 BOTTOM BRACKET	

foundation of a bicycle. It's the part that connects everything else together. Without a good frame, regardless of the components used to make it a complete bicycle, it will always be less than satisfactory. On the other hand, start with a good frame and improvements are generally relatively easy. Better components can be added right away or later.

Figure 8-4 shows the parts of a frame. Frame sizes and shapes vary. Custom frames can be fitted to the rider, and stock manufactured frames come in a number of sizes. *Frame size* is the distance in inches from the center of the bottom bracket to the top of the seat-post tube. Many brands of bicycles offer sizes ranging from about 19 to 25 inches. Eventually, these sizes will probably all be in centimeters (metric system) in the United States, as is already the case in much of the world.

A range of from 19 to 25 inches will suit most teenagers and adults for exercise and physical fitness riding. Even when you consider bicycles designed for the same purposes, such as utility or touring, frame sizes and designs vary with the manufacturer. Oddball frame shapes have largely disappeared from the market, and the recent tendency is for even inexpensive bicycles to follow the basic design shapes of more expensive models. A certain frame size, however, as defined above, can still vary considerably in other dimensions from manufacturer to manufacturer.

One variable is the angle of the head and seat tubes, which are called the *frame angles* (Fig. 8-5). Generally, the angles of both the head and seat tubes on a bicycle are the same: that is, they are set parallel to each other. On general purpose and touring bicycles, the frame angles are generally about 72 degrees from the horizontal. Racing bicycles frequently use slightly greater angles—73 or 74 degrees.

Another important variable is the *reach*, the distance from saddle post to fork tube on the frame. The actual reach can be adjusted somewhat by using different length stems on handlebar posts, but you must have approximately the correct length top tube on the bicycle frame.

Still another variable is the size of the *rear triangle*. For general riding, touring, and especially for most types of racing, it's an advantage to have a short triangle so that the tire will be close to the seat tube. This gives a shorter wheel base and makes the frame more rigid.

Many inexpensive bicycles have large triangles. The longer chain and seat stays make the frame less rigid and subject to greater whip, an undesirable characteristic.

Desirable characteristics for a frame are light weight and a certain amount of rigidity. An extremely flexible frame wastes energy, while an extremely rigid frame is less comfortable. For general exercise and physical fitness riding, a happy medium is recommended. This will give both reasonable riding comfort and good control.

Making frames lighter while still giving them adequate strength and rigidity is an extremely complicated design problem. Unlike buying steak at the supermarket, lightweight bicycle frames generally costs more money than heavyweights.

Bicycle frames are made up of a series of tubes. The tubes used on inexpensive bicycles are commonly of seamed steel tubing, made by

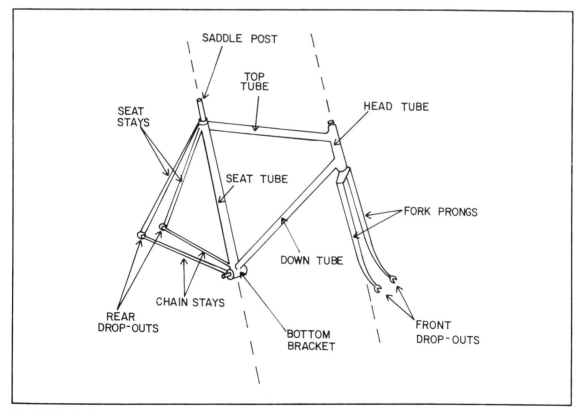

Fig. 8-5. Bicycle frame.

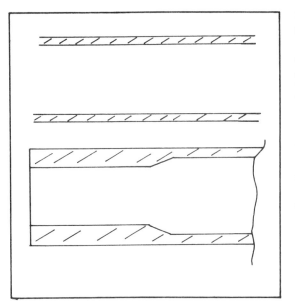

Fig. 8-6. Straight gauge tubing and butted tube with thicker gauge at one end.

wrapping a sheet of low-carbon steel into a tube and electrically welding it where the edges meet. This forms a straight-gauge tubing that is the same thickness the entire length.

Many bicycling authorities suggest that you forget about bicycle frames constructed of seamed low-carbon steel tubing. I don't completely agree with this. Low-carbon steel makes electric welding possible. The high heat caused by this inexpensive welding method would weaken a higher carbon steel, thus making possible inexpensive bicycles. These frames are often adequate for exercise and physical fitness riding and should be considered when cost is an important consideration.

The next step upward, and certainly much better, is seamless high-carbon tensile steel.

Since this tubing is stronger, thinner cross sections can be used to make a lighter frame.

The lowest cost frames of this material are straight-gauge. A butted-tube, which is gauge at one end is more expensive (Fig. 8-6). Double-butted (Fig. 8-7), which has a thicker gauge at both ends and a thinner gauge in the middle, is the most expensive.

The butting process is actually quite old. It was invented in 1897, by Alfred Reynolds, an English nailmaker. Over the years, the practicality of the tubing has been well demonstrated. Bicycle frames that use butted tubing are thicker on the ends where they join other tubes—the point where they are subjected to the greatest stress. The thinner gauge in the center where the strength is not needed allows a lighter weight frame.

When you look at a frame from the outside, you can't see the different gauges of wall thickness. The outside of the tubing is the same diameter throughout. The added thickness goes inward. Actually, it's difficult to observe even if you cut up the frame. The wall thickness of a top tube, for example, might be .022-inch in the middle and .032-inch at the ends. This is a difference of only about one-hundredth of an inch. Although the difference might appear slight or even unnoticeable to the eye, it makes for a much better bicycle frame. How do you know if the tubing is butted? You just have to take the manufacturer's word for it.

The next step upward in frame material is chrome-molybdenum (chrome-moly) or manganese-molybdenum steel. This tubing, like high-carbon steel seamless tubing, is available in straight-gauge, single-, and double-butted, constructions.

Reynolds 531 tubing is well known, but there are also many other top quality brands,

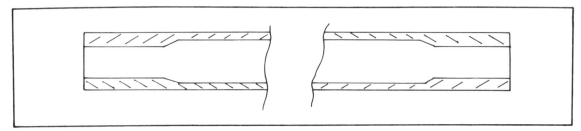

Fig. 8-7. Double-butted tube has thicker gauge at each end.

including Columbus, Falk, Super Vitus, and Champion. These will be indicated by stickers, usually placed on the seat tubes. The stickers will also tell you if the tubes are butted or double-butted.

Sometimes chrome-molybdenum or manganese-molybdenum steel is used only on the three main tubes, and less expensive tubing is used for the remainder of the frame. For example, the sticker might read "3 Chrome Molybdenum Main Tubes," which also indicates, since it is not mentioned, that the tubing is straight-gauge. If a manufacturer goes to the expense and trouble of using butted or double-butted tubing, you can be fairly sure that it will be indicated on the sticker.

The steel tubings described above—seamed low-carbon, seamless high-carbon, and chrome-molybdenum or manganese-molybdenum—must be joined together to form bicycle frames. Low-carbon steel can be welded and makes inexpensive bicycle frames possible. The high-carbon and alloy steels are generally assembled by low-heat brazing, because the high heat of welding would greatly weaken these types of steel. Not only that, but the weak point would be right at the joints where the strength is most needed. Brazing uses a brass or silver metal alloy filler. It can be done at about 1600°F or lower. This allows the tubes to be joined without seriously reducing their strength. Even with brazing, there is some loss in the tensile strength

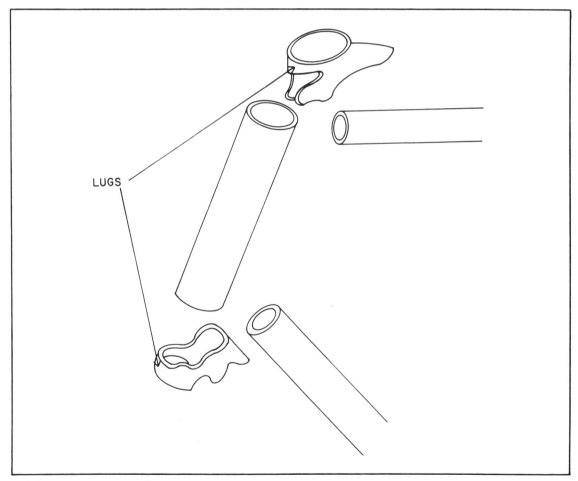

LUGS

Fig.8-8. Frame assembled with lugs.

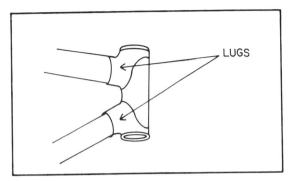

Fig. 8-9. Lugged frame assembly.

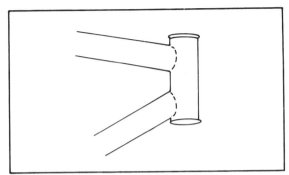

Fig. 8-11. Frame pieces are brazed or welded directly together.

of the tubing, but this can usually be kept within acceptable limits.

Frames are assembled with (Figs. 8-8 and 8-9) or without (Figs. 8-10 and 8-11) lugs. Frames without lugs are generally associated with inexpensive bicycles, but in fact many top quality frames are also made without lugs. Also, there is a growing tendency for cheap, poorly constructed frames to use lugs in an attempt to look like more expensive constructions.

The purpose of lugs is to strengthen joints by adding metal and distributing the stresses over larger areas. It's important, however, to have the ends of the tubes precision mitered. Lugs can and often are used to hide poorly fitted frame pieces. Lugs also perform a decorative function. They often have fancy cutouts and decorative shapes. On the other hand, a frame brazed together without lugs by a skilled craftsman can have an attractive appearance, too.

In comparison to welding, brazing is an expensive operation. It is difficult to absorb this cost on inexpensive frames. One method of cutting down on the cost is to use inexpensive brazing rod (filler) material. Unfortunately, this usually results in poorer bonding.

It is difficult for the novice—or almost anyone—to accurately judge the quality of brazing on a finished bicycle. This is especially true when lugs are used. In general, the best assurance of quality is a reputable manufacturer.

Drop-outs, the notched plates for the rear wheel axles (Fig. 8-12), are important frame

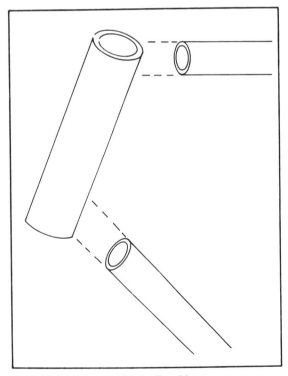

Fig. 8-10. Frame assembled without lugs.

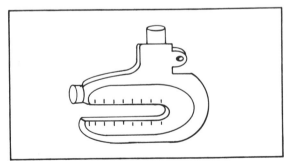

Fig. 8-12. Rear drop-out.

members. The cheaper ones are stamped out; the better ones are forged into shape.

The drop-outs on inexpensive bicycle frames are often installed by crimping them to the frame and then spot welding them. This is easily recognized by the breaks in the joints. This method has been widely criticized, but frames constructed in this manner will often pass quite stringent stress tests. In any case, in the lowest price range, there is little else available. More expensive frames generally have forged drop-outs that are brazed in place.

Forks are generally, although perhaps not technically, considered to be part of the bicycle frame. The *stem* is the part that passes through the head tube on the frame. The *blades* attach to the wheel. The blades normally curve forward about 2 inches from a straight line. This is called *rake*. Rake helps the bicycle to track in a straight line and to absorb road shock. Less rake results in quicker turning but poorer tracking.

The least expensive forks have flattened ends with notches for the axles. Better forks have drop-outs or fork-ends brazed or welded to the fork blades (Fig. 8-13). The cheapest of these are stamped construction. The best are forged into shape.

The drop-outs, or lack of them in the case of flattened and notched fork blades, can give a good indication of both the price and quality of a bicycle. From about the low end of the medium price range upward, most bicycles have forged drop-outs brazed or welded in place.

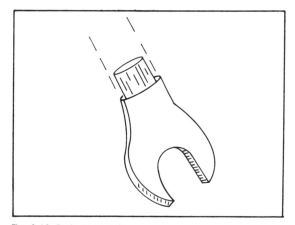

Fig. 8-13. Fork drop-out.

The closed triangle frames typically used on bicycles designed for boys and men results in a stronger and more rigid bicycle frame than do frames designed without a top frame tube for girls and women. There is a growing trend for women, especially for long distance touring and almost always for racing, to use bicycles with frames featuring top tubes, the same as men use. (The original reason for the design of women's bicycle frames without top tubes was to accommodate skirts while riding.)

For girls and women who still prefer a bicycle without the top tube, these will usually be satisfactory for exercise and physical fitness riding up to a moderate level of performance. The traditional design has two down tubes that run parallel to each other. A somewhat better arrangement is to have the upper tube joining the seat tube at a higher position. An even better arrangement is called the *mixte*. The bottom tube is the same as on a men's bicycle and two smaller tubes run in tandem from the top of the head tube to the drop-outs in the rear. While this construction still tends to have more undesirable whip than a similar men's frame, it is usually better than the other constructions described above.

Bicycle frames are also constructed of a variety of other materials, including stainless steel, aluminum, titanium, graphite, and plastics. Frames of these materials are generally more expensive and/or of unproven advantage for bicycle frames used for exercise and physical fitness riding.

Important frame variables include saddle tube length and angle, top tube length, frame height above ground, bracket height and wheel base (which is varied by length of stays), and angle and rake of front fork.

Bicycle frames are usually painted. This is both to protect the metal and for appearance. Chrome plating is used on the ends of the fork blades on some bikes, and in a few cases the entire frames are plated.

The quality of finishes applied by manufacturers vary greatly. When examining a new bicycle, make certain that there are no runs, chips, or other defects in the painted surface. These defects can indicate careless application by the manufacturers or careless handling of the bicycle. This type of damage often occurs during shipping and/or assembly of the bicycles. Some of this can be tolerated on inexpensive bicycles, but medium and high priced models should be closer to perfection.

Components

A bicycle is a frame plus its components. In general, better frames will feature better components, but there are some exceptions to this. The brand name of a particular bicycle is generally supplied by the frame manufacturer, but most often the components for completing the bicycle are from other manufacturers. The component parts often also have brands, and these are helpful in judging quality.

Bicycle components are frequently available in either steel or aluminum alloy. The main advantage of aluminum alloy is that it is lighter than steel; steel has the advantage of being less expensive. Both materials, when the components are properly designed and constructed, can give adequate strength. Bicycle components are also being made out of titanium and similar space-age materials, but these are generally too expensive for ordinary uses.

Hubs

There are two basic construction methods for making hubs. Inexpensive hubs are stamped out of steel. More expensive ones are precision machined out of steel or aluminum alloy. In addition to being as light in weight as possible, the hubs should rotate with as little friction as possible. This depends on a number of factors, especially the precision of the bearings and their housings.

The *flanges* are the parts of the hub that the spokes pass through. Hubs are made with both high and low flanges. Longer spokes are used with low flanges for better shock absorbing qualities than shorter spokes, and it makes them ideal for general riding and touring. High flanges use shorter spokes; this makes the wheel less springy and ideal for some types of racing.

Two basic methods are used to connect the axles to the bicycle frames: nuts on the ends of the threaded portion of the axles and quick-release devices. The latter have a quick-release skewer that passes through a hollow axle. A lever on one end locks both sides of the axle in the drop-outs.

The quick-release-type are generally associated with higher priced bicycles. Another method for removing a wheel without tools is to replace the axle nuts with wing nuts and some manufactured bicycles come with these (Fig. 8-14).

The advantages of quick wheel removal without tools is sometimes offset by the fact that it makes stealing wheels easier.

The quick release hubs were originally designed for racing, where quick wheel changing is essential. These devices are now found on many medium priced and most expensive touring bicycles, however.

Most hubs, except those with internal gear or coaster brakes, are packed with grease. Internal gear and coaster brake hubs typically use oil. A few other types of hubs, including some expensive racing models, also use oil. Two basic types of bearings used are *caged* (in retainers) and *loose*. There was a time when inexpensive hubs had bearings in retainers, and more expensive ones were loose. While this is still generally true, there is a trend toward expensive hubs using bearings in retainers, too. Needless to say, this greatly simplifies lubricating and overhauling.

Permanently sealed bearings eliminate not only the need for periodic lubrication, but also the touchy problem of adjusting cones against the bearings. Several brands are now on the market. Once on the bike, they require no maintenance. A drawback is that these hubs are very expensive, although cheaper versions are now being manufactured and used on more and more bicycles.

Permanently sealed bearings are also being used in other parts of bicycles. My guess is that they will become less expensive and make the old style bicycle bearings largely obsolete. Even at present prices, I consider them well worth the price for use on medium and high priced bicycles.

Another hub variable is the number of spoke holes. These must match the number on the rim. Many hubs have 36 spoke holes, and

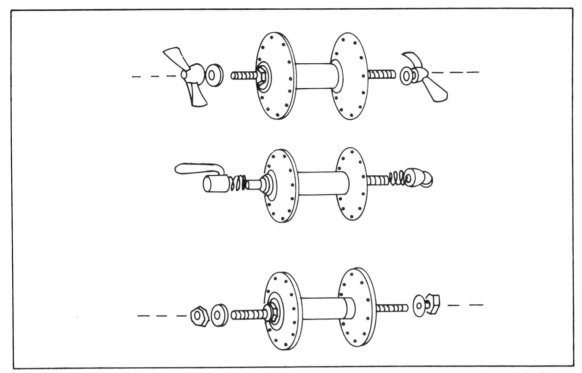

Fig. 8-14. Axle connected to frame by means of nuts (top), quick release devices (center), and wing nuts (bottom).

these work well for exercise and physical fitness riding.

Rims

There are two basic types of rims: those for *clincher* tires (Fig. 8-15) and those for *tubular* tires (Fig. 8-16). Clincher tires have beads that are held in place on the rim by lips, and tubular tires are glued to the rims. Clincher rims are available in steel and more expensive but lighter weight aluminum alloy. Most tubular rims are of aluminum alloy. Some tubular rims are filled with wood or plastic inserts to reinforce the otherwise hollow area.

For general exercise and physical fitness riding, I suggest that you use clincher rims. These are less expensive, and you have the

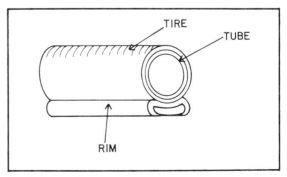

Fig. 8-15. Clincher.

Fig. 8-16. Tubular.

advantage of not having to sew up the tires, as is necessary on the tubular rims.

Spokes

Spokes are available in straight-gauge and butted (Fig. 8-17). The butted ones are of larger diameter on the ends than in the middle. Unlike butted bicycle frames, you can see this feature on spokes.

Spokes are made from aluminum, steel, and stainless steel. For general riding, I prefer stainless steel spokes, because they look better than the aluminum or regular steel ones. The aluminum spokes have the advantage of lighter weight.

When a hub is spoked or *laced* to a rim, various lacing patterns can be used. A three cross pattern is typical for touring bicycles. Special spoking patterns that give stiffer wheels are frequently used on some types of racing bicycles, but these are usually unnecessary for typical exercise and fitness riding.

TIRES

The two main types bicycle tires are clinchers (or wired-ons) that use inner tubes and tubulars (or sew-ups). Tubeless tires were used commonly on bicycles, but they are rare today.

Tubulars are called sew-ups because the inner tubes are actually sewn inside the tire with a needle and thread. Repair requires considerable skill and patience. Tubulars are glued to the rim or attached with a sticky tape.

Clincher tires have wire beads at each edge of the casing where it goes over the rim. They are generally heavier than tubulars. This heavier

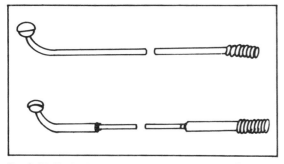

Fig. 8-17. Straight gauge spoke and butted spoke.

weight is a disadvantage, because the rolling resistance is greater. For general exercise and physical fitness riding, however, there are a number of advantages that help to offset the weight disadvantage. Clinchers are generally more puncture resistant, give better traction in wet conditions, have a longer useful life, and allow easier repair of punctures. Clinchers generally have lower maximum inflation pressures than tubulars, because it's the tire and not the tube that determines the maximum pressure. Typical clinchers used on narrow 26-inch and 27-inch wheels have a maximum pressure of 60 to 75 pounds (p.s.i.), although some models are on the market that take up to 90 pounds or more. Higher pressures are an advantage in decreasing rolling resistance, but they make for a bumpy ride, especially on a bicycle with a stiff frame.

While most clincher tires cannot be folded to make carrying a spare easy on long rides, some models are now available that can be folded.

Balloon tires, with 1½-inch cross section or more, have more rolling resistance than a narrow tire, such as those used on lightweight bicycles.

Tubulars have several advantages over clinchers. They are lighter: racing models weigh about 7½ ounces with inner tubes and touring models about 12 ounces with inner tubes. For a clincher tube and tire combination, most weight at least 17 ounces and many considerably more than this. Tubulars generally have higher maximum pressures than do clinchers. Some tubulars used for track racing bicycles use 140 pounds or more, but 100 pounds is a more typical figure for touring-type. Tubulars have less tread on the ground than do clinchers, therefore, they give less rolling resistance, but also less traction.

Disadvantages of tubulars as compared to clinchers are that they are more easily worn out and punctured and that they are more time consuming to repair. Several spares with inner tubes already sewn in place will fit under a bicycle saddle, however. In general, tubulars are more expensive than clinchers, although there is some overlapping in prices between the more expensive clinchers and the less expensive tubulars.

Tubulars usually come with a European-type valve called the *Presta valve*. To inflate with a service station air supply or a common hand pump, a special adapter is required. These are inexpensive and readily available at bike shops, or you can buy the type of bicycle pump that will fit the *Presta* valve.

Clinchers use a different type of rim than tubulars, so the tires aren't interchangeable. Generally, inexpensive bicycles and higher medium priced ones will have clinchers, which are probably more suitable for these bicycles anyway. To switch over to tubulars involves lacing different type rims to the hubs, which is a fairly costly and involved operation.

Some bicycles in the upper-medium price range have tubulars, and they are quite common on expensive bicycles. I believe that it is best to start out with clinchers for general exercise and physical fitness riding. It seems to me that tubulars are only worth the extra trouble if you have a real need for the extra performance for racing or long distance riding.

Flat tires are probably the biggest single problem faced by bicycle owners and riders. While the particular tire will have varying degrees of puncture resistance, many attempts have been made to go beyond this. One method is to add a liquid sealant to the inside of the inner tube. These sealants are readily available from bicycle shops.

Another puncture-proofing method is to fill the inner tubes with materials that trap air into tiny pockets. There has been some success with this, but present methods add considerable weight to the tires—undesirable from a performance standpoint.

A third method is to use latex inner tubes. These are so elastic that it is difficult for even a sharp object to penetrate them. Several brands are now on the market, and they do not add extra weight to the wheels.

Wheels

Bicycle wheels are the sum of the hub, spokes, rim, tire, inner tube, and rim liners. A lightweight, narrow, high pressure wheel is a tremendous advantage in overcoming rolling resistance. Larger wheels, up to about 27 inches or 28 inches in diameter, are also an advantage.

Wheels on new bicycles have varying degrees of *trueness*. For a rough check of the trueness of wheels in bicycle showrooms, spin the wheels and use the caliper brake pads or the flat eraser end of a pencil as a guide to check trueness. In this manner, any serious deviations can be noted. Have the dealer make any required corrections before you buy the bicycle. Spoke plucking, like kicking a tire on a used car, generally has little or no value.

Saddles and Saddle Posts

Type, shape, quality, and price are all considerations. A comfortable saddle can make considerable difference in the enjoyment of exercise and physical fitness cycling.

The least expensive saddles typically have metal bases, some padding, and thin plastic covers or padding as part of a molded rubber or plastic cover. A slightly more expensive type has a contour shaped base of flexible nylon or plastic covered with leather or plastic materials. Depending on design and construction, these are available from fairly inexpensive to very expensive models, and have, to a large extent, replaced the old standard leather racing and touring saddles. The leather ones, however, including hand worked ones, are still around. There are also a few people still around who think these are the best.

Leather saddles generally have to be broken in. This means some uncomfortable riding until either the saddle changes shape or the rider adjusts to the shape of the saddle. My own experience with leather saddles is that neither of these things ever happen.

Bicycle saddles are now made out of new "slow memory" foam materials. These saddles are advertised as being much more comfortable than regular bicycle saddles.

It's important that the angle of the saddle be adjustable. This might be part of the saddle post or saddle attachment bracket. Some of the better saddle posts feature continuous micro-adjustment capabilities. Less expensive ones, but still satisfactory for most purposes, can be positioned only in notches and not between them. The difference is very subtle, however. While it might make the fraction of a second difference in

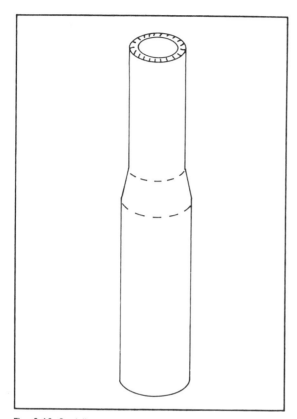

Fig. 8-18. Saddle post.

winning or losing a race, it probably would not be worth the extra cost for ordinary exercise and physical fitness riding. More expensive saddles often have a means of adjusting the tension to make the saddle stiffer or more flexible.

Give careful consideration to the quality of the saddle. Some saddles will wear quickly. On others, molded plastic or rubber covers can be replaced when they wear out. Still other saddles cannot be recovered so easily and will usually have to be replaced completely.

Important factors to keep in mind when selecting a saddle are:

—Suitability for your needs, especially for comfort and riding efficiency.

—Quality, especially as it pertains to durability.

—Price, which must be weighed carefully against the other factors.

When you are selecting a new bicycle, many dealers will make saddle switches to make a sale.

This can often be used as leverage in getting exactly what you want.

Saddle posts (Fig. 8-18) are also important. Inexpensive saddle posts are often made of steel. Lighter and more expensive ones are aluminum alloy. Make certain that the saddle post is long enough so that at least several inches will extend down into the seat tube at the highest adjustment that will be used.

Handlebars

Handlebars are available in a variety of configurations. The three basic types are flat, raised, and dropped. The flat and raised types allow you to ride in an upright position. This allows for better vision when riding in traffic. Older riders and riders with low agility levels often find these handlebars suitable to their needs. Within the flat and raised types are many variations.

To the novice eye, dropped handlebars may all look alike, but there are actually many variations. The choice depends both on individual preference and intended use of the bicycle. Some offer more hand positions than others, and those that allow the most variation are convenient for exercise and physical fitness riding.

Handlebars are made from both steel and aluminum alloy. Flat and raised handlebars are typically made of steel; the dropped type are available in both steel and alloy. In the general line of bicycles, the alloy is typically found only on the more expensive models, usually starting around the middle of the medium-price range.

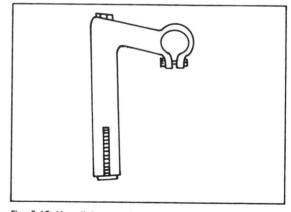

Fig. 8-19. Handlebar post.

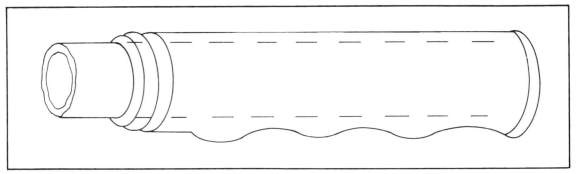

Fig. 8-20. Handlebar grip.

Steel is stronger, and for this reason there are expensive steel handlebars designed for track racing bicycles that can take tremendous forces.

Handlebar Posts

Handlebar posts (Fig. 8-19) are also called *stems* and *goosenecks*. They attach inside the fork tube or stem that passes through the head tube of the bicycle frame. The handlebar post is held inside the fork stem by means of an expansion device. The cheaper bikes have an expansion device on one side and a regular protruding bolt head. More expensive bikes have double expansion and either a regular protruding bolt head or an Allen nut for a neater appearance, but many bicycle mechanics prefer the bolt head because it is easier to secure.

Handlebar posts are available in steel and aluminum alloy. The latter is lighter and generally more expensive. The handlebar posts have various configurations, which have a bearing on both the height and distance forward of the handlebars on the bicycle. The height can generally be adjusted within a certain range. It is important to have at least 1½ inches of the post down inside the fork tube. Forward/backward adjustments usually require switching to another handlebar post with a different length neck, but there are also a few handlebar posts on the market that allow forward/backward adjustment.

Grips and Taping

Rubber or plastic grips (Fig. 8-20) are generally used on flat and raised handlebars. In addition to better appearance, they also provide for a better grip, help absorb road shock, and provide protection from injury by covering the ends of the handlebars.

Taping (Fig. 8-21) is generally used in place of grips on dropped handlebars. With some exceptions, plastic tape is the standard for inexpensive bicycles and cloth for medium priced and expensive models. Padded tape is also available. This will help to absorb road shock. Cycling gloves can also be used for the same purpose. The ends of the handlebars should always be plugged. This is not only for holding the ends of the tape in place, but also for safety.

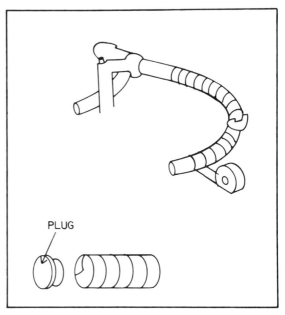

Fig. 8-21. Handlebar taping. Plug is used for holding tape in place.

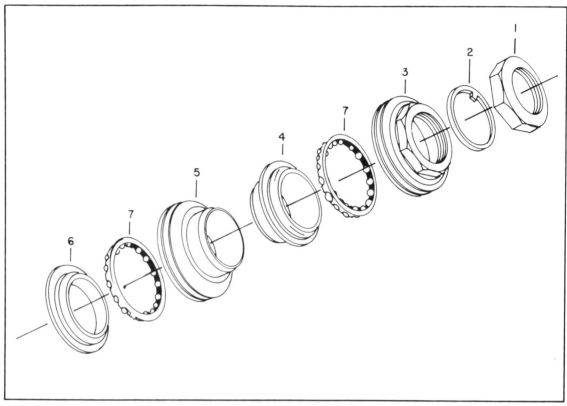

Fig. 8-22. Headset consists of (1) locknut, (2) lock washer, (3) adjusting cup, (4) upper stationary cone, (5) lower stationary cone, (6) crown cone, and (7) ball retainer.

Headsets

The headset (Fig. 8-22) consists of the bearings, cups, cones, and other parts that allow the fork to turn in the head tube of the bicycle frame (Fig. 8-23). When inspecting a bicycle, check to make sure that the fork turns freely and smoothly in the head tube. Since the parts that count are inside where you can't see them without disassembling the headset, it's usually necessary to assume that they are of a quality in keeping with the rest of the bicycle. Headsets are generally a fairly trouble-free part of a bicycle.

Brakes

Coaster brakes (Fig. 8-24) operate by back pedaling. They are commonly used on single-speed bicycles and sometimes on hub-geared models. These brakes vary in design, quality, and price, but most will give good service.

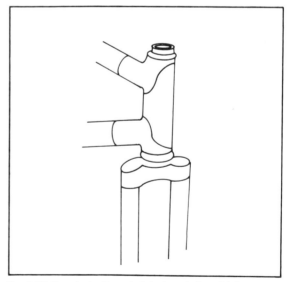

Fig. 8-23. Headset allows fork to turn in head tube.

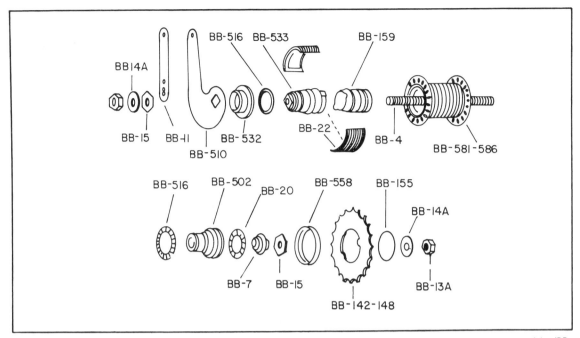

Fig. 8-24. Bendix Model 70 coaster brake. Parts are: (BB-4) axle, (BB-7) adjusting cone, (BB-11) arm clip assembly, (BB-13A) axle nut, (BB-14A) axle washer, (BB-15) lock nut, (BB-20) retainer, (BB-22) sub-assembly, (BB-502) drive screw, (BB-510) brake arm, (BB-516) retainer, (BB-532) dust cap, (BB-533) expander, (BB-558) dust cap, and (BB-581-586) hub shell.

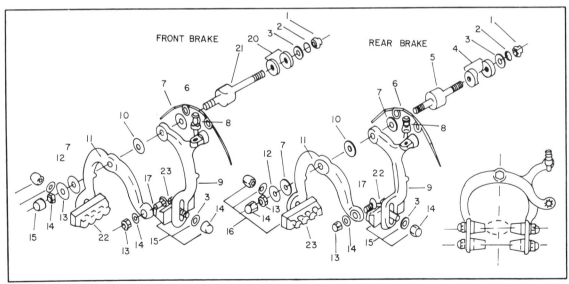

Fig. 8-25. Side-pull caliper brakes. Parts are: (1) lock nut for pivot bolt, (2) toothed lock washer, (3) washer A, (4) radius bushing—front, (5) pivot bolt—front, (6) arm return spring, (7) arm washer, (8) cable adjusting barrel and nut, (9) brake arm Y-shape, (10) arm spacer, (11) brake arm C-shape, (12) washer C, (13) lock nut, (14) cap nut, (15) brake shoe complete—right, (16) brake shoe complete—left, (17) cable anchor bolt, (18) washer B, (19) cap nut, (2) radius bushing—rear, (21) pivot bolt—rear, (22) brake shoe—right, and (23) brake shoe left.

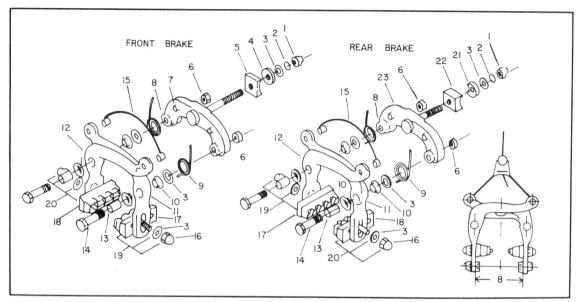

Fig. 8-26. Center-pull caliper brakes. Parts are: (1) lock nut, (2) lock washer, (3) washer, (4) radius bushing—front, (5) square seating pad—front, (6) lock nut for pivot bolt, (7) arm bridge with center bolt, (8) LH arm return spring, (9) RH arm return spring, (10) flanged thrust washer, (11) inner brake arm, (12) outer brake arm, (13) bushing, (14) pivot bolt, (15) center cable, (16) cap nut for brake shoe, (17) brake shoe—left, (18) brake shoe—right, (19) brake shoe complete—left, (20) brake shoe complete—right, (21) radius bushing—rear, (22) square seating pad—rear, and (23) arm bridge with center bolt.

Caliper brakes are often used on hub-geared bicycles and on the majority of derailleur-geared bicycles. Caliper brakes are operated by hand levers that press rubber pads against the sides of the rim. The two main types in use are *side-pull* (Fig. 8-25) and *center-pull* (Fig. 8-26). The side-pull type are commonly thought of as being inferior, probably because poorly designed and

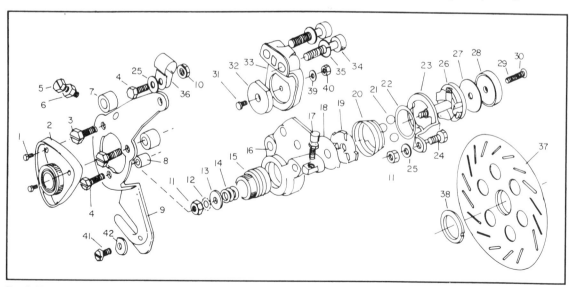

Fig. 8-27. Disk brake.

constructed models are often used on cheap bicycles. Some of the finest and most expensive brakes made, however, such as the Campagnolo and Zeus brands, are side-pull. As far as caliper brakes go, on most inexpensive and medium priced bicycles the center-pull models generally seem more satisfactory.

Both center-pull and side-pull brakes have two arms that rotate in opposite directions to form clamps. These clamps are the rubber pads that fit against the rims. The pivot on side-pulls is at one point at the side. Center-pulls have a separate pivot point for each arm. They have a transverse crossover cable with a sliding device to which a single wire connects and goes to the control levers.

Some caliper brakes have quick release levers that make wheel removal easier. Another feature to look for is a cable adjuster to take up slack in the cable.

When checking caliper brakes on a particular bicycle, make sure that they spring back quickly when the hand lever is released. Weak spring action is a common problem with caliper brakes, especially with low cost models.

In use, caliper brakes tend to work poorly in wet weather and on downhill runs. For this reason and others, *disk brakes* (Fig. 8-27) are growing in popularity, and some stock bicycles now come with these. The better designs are not affected when they get wet and the cooling is better than on brake-pad models. Disk brakes, however, tend to be heavy, somewhat complicated, and expensive in comparison to the brake-pad type.

Drum brakes are another possibility, but although these are available, they do not seem to be very popular on regular bicycles. Their primary use seems to be when extra heavy-duty braking is required, such as on tandem bicycles.

Pedals

The least expensive pedals cannot be dismantled for lubrication or overhaul. These are available with metal bases and rubber foot pads, or all-metal construction. This type of pedal is usually found only on the least expensive manufactured bicycles. They generally lack precision and are subject to frequent breakdowns. The advantage is the low cost.

Pedals with metal bases and rubber foot pads that can be disassembled for repair and lubrication are usually of better quality. They are popular for use on utility bicycles. The rubber foot pads can be an advantage over all metal pedals for riding with thin soled shoes.

Toe clips and straps will not ordinarily attach to the rubber pedals, but there are a few pedals of this type that come with clips, straps, or both. The use, advantages, and disadvantages of clips and straps are detailed later in this chapter.

Metal pedals are called *rattraps* and can be used with or without toe clips or straps. Most of the metal pedals have teeth to keep your shoes from slipping. Racing pedals, however, generally have no teeth. Special shoes with cleats are worn to hold your feet in position on the pedals.

Regardless of the type of pedals, they should spin freely. Most standard pedals are lubricated with grease. Pedals with permanenently sealed bearings are also on the market now. Some top quality racing pedals are lubricated with oil. As a general rule, the more expensive the pedals, the lighter they are in weight.

Crank Sets

A *crank set* consists of the bottom bracket bearings and assembly and the cranks. The two basic types of cranks are one-piece and three-piece arrangements making up the pedal cranks and axle.

The one-piece-type (Fig. 8-28) is frequently used on inexpensive bicycles and less frequently on medium-priced ones. These are made of steel: they are strong and relatively trouble free. The main disadvantage is extra weight, but this should not be much of a problem for general exercise and physical fitness riding.

The three-piece-type are made up of an axle and two separate crank arms. There are two basic methods of attaching the crank arms to the axle: with *cotters* (called *cottered cranks*; Fig. 8-29) and with bolts that hold the crank arms on wedged axle ends (called *cotterless*; Fig. 8-30). The axles on both types are typically made of steel: cottered cranks are generally steel and cotterless are usually of aluminum alloy.

Cotterless cranks, used mainly on expensive bicycles when they were first introduced, are

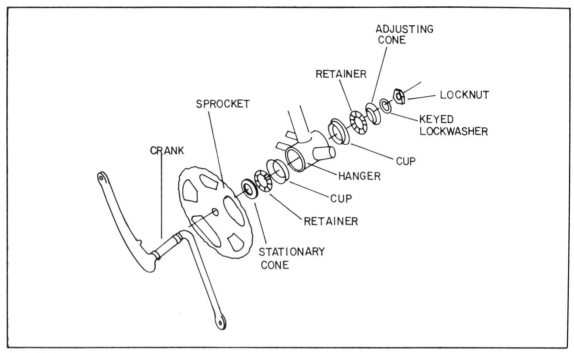

Fig. 8-28. One-piece crank set.

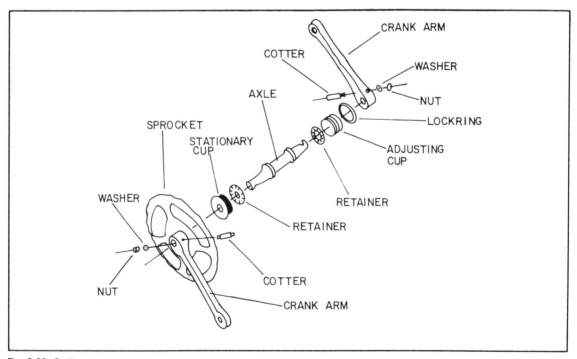

Fig. 8-29. Cottered crank set.

186

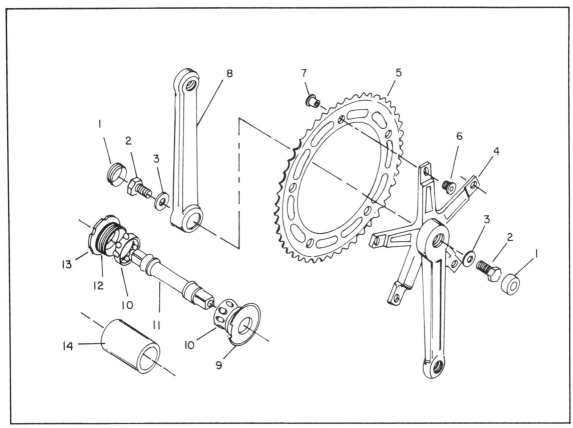

Fig. 8-30. Cotterless crank set. Parts are: (1) crank arm dust cap, (2) spindle bolt, (3) spindle washer, (4) right crank arm, (5) chainwheel, (6) chainwheel fixing bolt, (7) chainwheel fixing nut, (8) left crank arm, (9) RH fixed cup, (10) steel ball retainer for bottom bracket, (11) bottom bracket spindle, (12) LH adjustable cup, (13) lock ring, and (14) dust seal.

rapidly replacing the cottered-type at all price levels.

For the general run of stock bicycles, the length of crank arms is fairly standardized, but there are some variations. Longer arms can give better leverage for increased riding efficiency, but there must be adequate ground clearance for safe riding and cornering.

With the chain removed, the crank assembly should spin freely, with no noise. Most crank assemblies have bearings that are either in retainers or loose, and some quality bicycles now feature permanently sealed bearings. Other manufacturers will probably be switching to these. The advantage of not having to overhaul (clean and lubricate) the bottom bracket assembly can be worth the additional cost for many riders.

Chains

Chains are an extremely important part of a bicycle, but it takes a very experienced person to even begin to judge the quality of chains just by looking at them. In most cases, you will have to assume that the chain used on a particular bicycle is of a quality in keeping with the rest of the bike. Most makers of quality bicycles do not skimp on the chains used.

Control Cables

Control cables are used for caliper and disk brakes and shifters. The cables should move freely through the housings. Inexpensive bicycles usually have cables inside housings for their entire length. More expensive bicycles often have those sections of cable that run parallel to the frame tubes outside the housings to reduce friction. The cable housings on inexpensive bicycles are typically held to the frames by clamps, and more expensive bicycles often feature lugs that are brazed to the bicycle frames.

UNDERSTANDING GEARS

The remainder of the components that go to make up a complete bicycle—chainwheels, rear sprockets, freewheels, shifters, and controls—are best covered along with their operation. When selecting gears, not only quality must be considered, but also type, number of gears, and gear ratios.

Fixed-Sprocket Track Bicycles

Perhaps the best way to gain a basic understanding of gearing systems and gear ratios is to begin with a discussion of a track racing bicycle with a fixed-sprocket (non-freewheeling) rear hub (Fig. 8-31). With this arrangement, when the wheel turns, the chainwheel and cranks also turn.

The beauty of this system is its simplicity: if both the rear sprocket and chainwheel are the same size and have the same number of teeth, the gear ratio is one-to-one (1:1). Some small sprockets have only every other tooth, but in computing gear ratios, the missing teeth are counted as though they were there. One-to-one is an extremely low gear ratio—the bicycle would be easy to pedal, but you would not go very far

with each pedal cycle. A more common arrangement is with the chainwheel larger than the rear sprocket. This makes the bicycle harder to pedal, but you go further with each pedal cycle. The formula for determining the gear ratio is: Gear Ratio = Number of teeth on chainwheel divided by Number of teeth on rear sprocket. If, for example, there are 45 teeth on the chainwheel and 15 on the rear sprocket, the gear ratio is 45 divided by 15 or three-to-one (3:1).

In actual practice, *gear values* rather than gear ratios are generally used. The formula for determining gear value is: Gear Value = Gear ratio × Wheel diameter. If, for example, the chainwheel has 48 teeth and the rear sprocket 14 teeth, the gear ratio, rounded off to the nearest tenth, is 3.4. The gear value is 3.4 × 27, or 91.8. The gear value represents the size the wheel would be on a direct drive (non-freewheeling) bicycle with a one-to-one gear ratio. In this example, the wheel would be 91.8 inches in diameter.

Notice, however, that this is not the distance covered. To compute the distance covered, multiply the gear value by 3.14. Since multiplying by a constant only serves to increase the size of the numbers, however, gear values rather than distance covered are usually used.

Single-Speed Bicycles

The drive assembly of a regular single-speed bicycle, unlike the track hub described above, will coast or freewheel when the pedals are

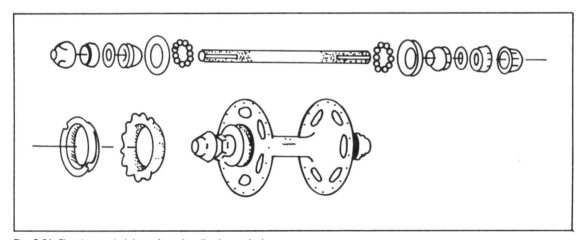

Fig. 8-31. Fixed-sprocket (non-freewheeling) rear hub.

stationary. This is accomplished by a freewheeling mechanism between the rear sprocket and the rear hub. The rear wheel cannot turn slower than the rear sprocket is turning, but it can rotate faster.

To calculate gear values, disregard coasting and use the same formula as for the fixed-sprocket hub.

While you have only a single gear value on a single-speed bicycle, you do have a choice of what that value is in the sense that you can change to sprockets with different numbers of teeth to obtain a new gear value. While a track bicycle will often have a gear value of 90 or higher, for ordinary exercise and physical fitness riding a gear value of about 60 to 80 would be about right.

Hub-Geared Bicycles

Hub-geared bicycles allow you to switch into two or more different gear ratios while riding. On a three-speed, which is the most common number used on hub-geared bicycles, the gear shifting is usually done by a lever or twist grip. There is a set position for each gear, typically marked L for low gear, N for neutral or sprocket gear ratio, and H for high gear.

The gear value for the N position can be determined by counting the teeth on the rear sprocket and chainwheel and then making the calculations as though the bicycle were a single-speed. The other two gear values can be determined only with difficulty, but the manufacturer usually includes these in the specifications. A sprocket or chainwheel switch to one with a different number of teeth will change all three gear values. For example, one make of three-speed hub has a 48-tooth chainwheel and a 14-tooth rear sprocket. The gear values of L, N, and H are 68, 88, and 120 respectively. This is an extremely high range of values for a three-speed. With a 16-tooth rear sprocket, the same setup would have gear values of 60, 78, and 104. This would be about right for exercise and physical fitness riding for a person who is already in fairly good shape. A 19-tooth rear sprocket gives gear values of 49, 66, and 88. This is a fairly low range of gears and would be about right for a person with a low endurance level who is starting out on an exercise program.

At various times, internal-geared hubs with automatic shiftings have been introduced on the market. The idea sounds good: you pedal and the bicycle automatically changes to the correct gear ratio. These have never become very popular, though, perhaps because they have never been perfected.

Derailleur-Geared Bicycles

You can study the operation of derailleur gears by placing the bicycle in a maintenance rack or upside down so that the pedals can be rotated and the shift levers operated. Countertop demonstrators that many bicycle shops have to acquaint potential customers with derailleur mechanisms will serve the same purpose.

First, consider a five-speed. This has a cluster of five sprockets at the rear hub, each with a different number of teeth. As was the case with the single-speed, there is a freewheeling mechanism between the sprocket cluster and the hub. There is a single chainwheel at the crank. The gear values will depend on which of the rear sprockets the chain is on. There will be five different gear values. For example, if the chainwheel has 50 teeth and the rear cluster from the largest inside sprocket outward have 28, 24, 20, 17, and 14, the gear values from the lowest (the 28-tooth sprocket) to the highest would be 48, 56, 68, 80, and 96.

In order for the system to work, the chain must be moved from one rear sprocket to another. The chain is actually derailed from one sprocket so that it will move over onto the next one. With a five-speed mounted so that the derailleur can be operated by hand, turn the pedals and then operate the shift lever. If a 10-speed bicycle is used for the demonstration, simply leave the front derailleur in either position and work only the control lever for the rear derailleur. (On the five-speed, there is only one derailleur control lever.)

Notice that the rear derailleur mechanism (Fig. 8-32) performs two basic functions: it moves the chain from sprocket to sprocket, and it takes up the slack in the chain. The latter is necessary, as without this feature the chain tension would be different on each sprocket. On a single-speed bicycle, a single chain length

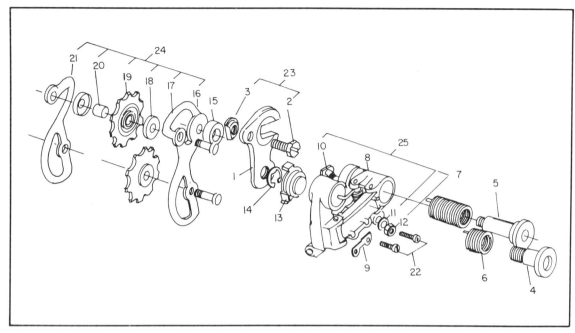

Fig. 8-32. Rear derailleur. Parts are: (1) adapter, (2) adapter screw, (3) adapter nut, (4) adapter mounting bolt, (5) plate mounting bolt, (6) B-tension spring, (7) P-tension spring, (8) mechanism assembly, (9) adjusting plate, (10) cable fixing bolt, (11) cable fixing washer, (12) cable fixing nut, (13) adapter bushing, (14) stop ring, (15) plate bushing, (16) pulley bolt, (17) inner cage plate, (18) pulley cap, (19) pulley, (20) pulley bushing, (21) outer cage plate, (22) adjusting screw, (23) adapter screw and nut, (24) pulley plate assembly, and (25) cable fixing set.

suffices. On the derailleur system, many lengths are needed.

The rear derailleur mechanism has two small pulleys with cages around them that move inward and outward by means of transversing arms that are shaped in a parallelogram under spring tension. The cage remains parallel to the sprockets. (A few new designs vary slightly from this.) The inward travel is by means of an operating shift lever and outward by action of a spring mechanism when the tension on the control lever is released. The chain is derailed only from one sprocket to the next. Skipping sprockets when you shift is poor technique and damages chain and sprockets. The chain must be moving, that is, the bicycle pedaled, for shifting to take place.

The pulley cage is also under spring tension toward the rear of the bicycle. This keeps the spring in tension regardless of which front chainwheel and rear sprocket the chain is on.

The shift operating mechanism on most derailleur systems is continuous action. There are no set stops for each gear. The cable pulls the parallelogram open and shifts the derailleur mechanism toward the high side (largest sprocket but lowest gear). Release the tension on the cable, and a spring returns the mechanism to the low side (smallest sprocket but highest gear). Only the limits are adjustable. There are two adjustment screws: one limits the pulley travel on the high side, and the other limits the pulley travel on the low side. These are usually marked by the adjusting screws with an H for high side and an L for low side.

The pulley that derails the chain is called the *jockey wheel* or *roller*. The lower roller, which maintains the chain tension, is called the *tension wheel* or *roller*. The rear sprocket cluster is often called the *freewheel*. The hub of the sprocket contains the freewheeling mechanism.

Five-sprocket rear clusters have become the standard number, but other numbers, especially three and six, are sometimes used.

The five-speed derailleur system described above is made into a 10-speed by means of a double chainwheel at the crank, and into a 15-speed by means of a triple chainwheel at the crank and separate front derailleur systems with their own control levers.

A front derailleur mechanism (Fig. 8-33) derails the chain, causing it to move from one sprocket to the next in a manner similar to the rear derailleur. The front mechanism does not have a device for maintaining chain tension, however. This is taken care of by the rear tension device.

Like the rear derailleur, the front derailleur is cable operated and has two limit adjusting screws. The small inside-located chainwheel gives the lower gear, and the larger outside-located chainwheel gives the higher gear. This is exactly the opposite of the rear sprockets.

On most front derailleurs, the lever pull deforms the parallelogram of the pantograph outward, moving the chain from the smaller to the larger chainwheel. The spring action when the tension on the lever is released pulls the parallelogram inward. A problem with this arrangement is that pulling the rear control lever toward you gives a lower gear, but pulling the front control lever toward you gives a higher gear. It takes considerable practice to get used to this.

A few models of front derailleurs work opposite this: the spring moves the cage outward, and the lever pulls it inward. This simplifies the operation in that pulling either control lever toward you always results in a lower gear, and pushing either control lever away from you always results in a higher gear, that is, until the limits are reached.

A major problem in "selling" the derailleur system is the amount of skill required to operate it. On most derailleurs, the shifting must be done by feel, as there are no set positions for

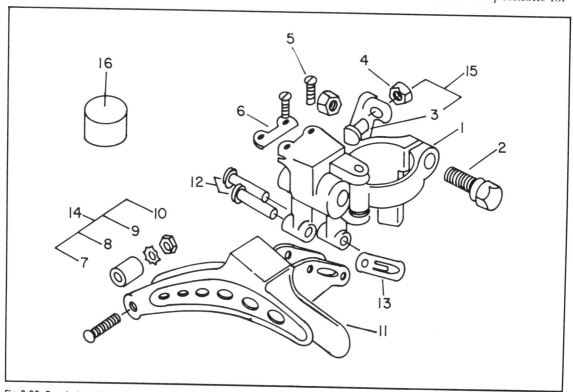

Fig.8-33. Front derailleur. Parts are: (1) mechanism unit, (2) clamp bolt, (3) cable fixing bolt, (4) cable fixing nut, (5) adjusting bolt, (6) adjusting plate, (7) chain guide spacer bolt, (8) chain guide spacer, (9) toothed lock washer, (10) nut, (11) chain guide, (12) pin A, (13) clip A, (14) chain guide spacer and bolt set, (15) cable fixing bolt and nut set, and (16) bushing.

centering the chain over individual sprockets.

There have been numerous attempts to get around this problem, such as positive indexing mechanisms with two control cables and free-wheeling at the chainwheel, which allows shifting even when the rider is not pedaling. The continuous lever systems remain the most common, however.

Regardless of whether you decide on a 5-speed, 10-speed, or 15-speed derailleur system, you will want to consider carefully what the gear values will be. Most new bicycles come with a gear chart showing the gear values for the particular rear sprockets and chainwheels used. If not, you can count the sprocket teeth and calculate them. A typical chart is as follows:

Teeth on Rear Sprockets

		34	28	22	18	14	
Teeth on	46	37	44	57	69	89	Gear
Chainwheel	52	41	50	64	78	100	Values

The gear development, the gear values from the lowest to the highest, is 37, 41, 44, 50, 57, 64, 69, 78, 89, and 100. This is a fairly wide range of gears that would serve well for many types of exercise and physical fitness riding. Not all rear derailleurs will handle a range of from 14 to 34 teeth sprockets, however. On road racing bicycles, a narrower range of gears is often used.

Here are a few points to keep in mind when selecting gear ratios:

- The weight of the bicycle is an important consideration. In general, a heavier bicycle should have a lower range of gear values than a lighter bicycle.
- If you will be riding in mountainous areas where there are a lot of steep hills, a lower range of gear values would be called for than if most of your riding is on level roads.
- Gear values over 100 are seldom required. The only way that most riders can handle these is by pedaling slowly. This is generally much less efficient than a lower gear value that can be handled at a higher cadence. A higher cadence is generally better for exercise and physical fitness riding.

- Try to get the gear values that you will be using the most in the middle of the gear range.

If you find a new bicycle that you like but with the wrong gear values for your purposes, you may be able to get the dealer to make sprocket switches and thereby change the gear values.

Location of shift levers is another important consideration. Early derailleur systems usually had the shift levers on the bottom tube. This is still the arrangement used for most racing bicycles. For touring and exercise riding, two other shift locations are also popular: on the handlebar stem and on the handlebar tips. Each location has its advantages and disadvantages, and the choice is an individual matter. It generally requires the most agility to handle the levers on the bottom tube, but this is considered the best location for high-speed riding.

Shift levers are sometimes located on the top tube, but for obvious reasons, this presents a safety hazard and I don't recommend them.

BICYCLE WEIGHT

It is one thing to consider the components that go to make up a bicycle and quite another to consider the assembled parts of an actual bicycle. You might have some choice in switching components, but this is usually limited, especially in the case of lower priced models.

If each component on one bicycle weighs just a little more than those on another bicycle, the total weight can be considerably more. That is why so much emphasis is placed on shaving off ounces on various components.

Price, design, quality, and weight are important factors to consider when selecting a bicycle. Most adult bicycles in the less than $150 price range will weigh 35 pounds or more—many will scale in at over 40 pounds. Most of this "extra" weight is a result of using less expensive materials and construction methods.

In the medium-price range of $150 to $250, most adult bicycles weigh from about 27 to 38 pounds. The lighter weights are usually at the high end of the price range. In this price range, some of the heavier bicycles do use the added weight to good advantage. When comparing a heavier bicycle with a lighter one, see how the extra weight has been used.

There is no getting around the fact that weight does affect performance, however. Eight pounds difference in the weight of two bicycles that are equal in all other respects will make a dramatic difference in ease of pedaling.

In the higher price ranges, you can expect lighter weight, usually under 30 pounds and frequently under 25, when you get to the $300 and over price tags.

THE RIDER AND THE BICYCLE

Charts have been developed for determining proper bicycle size from body measurements, but until you get to the stage where you want custom bicycles built for your body size, two simple measurements will usually suffice. The first is to take off your shoes and straddle over the frame bar with both feet flat on the floor. There should be at least ½-inch clearance between your crotch and the top frame tube. If there is more than 1-inch clearance, try the next larger frame size.

The second measurement is reach. This is the distance from the saddle to the handlebars. With your bent elbow placed against the forward end of the saddle, the extended fingers should reach to the center of the handlebar clamp. If this distance is off, minor corrections can be made by switching to a handlebar post with a different length neck. Also, adjustment can be made in the forward/backward adjustment of the saddle. For proper balance, the forward tip of the saddle should generally be about 2 inches behind the crank axle center.

ACCESSORIES

You won't need much extra equipment on a bicycle for exercise and physical fitness riding, so consider extra equipment only in terms of what you need and what isn't included with the bicycle you choose. It's not economical to purchase a bicycle with accessories you don't want. Sometimes a dealer will take these off and reduce the price accordingly or exchange them for spare parts like spare tires and tubes that you will need in the future.

Typical accessories include fenders, kick stands, chain guards, carrying racks, lights, reflectors, tire pumps, water bottles, and tool kits. As a general rule, it is best to purchase accessories that are approximately of the same general quality as the bicycle.

Since accessories add weight to bicycles, it's important to decide if the compromise in weight versus usefulness makes it worthwhile to add a particular accessory.

LEARNING TO RIDE

Although most of us learned to ride bikes when we were young, some adults may have to learn first.

You can, of course, learn to ride a bicycle without ever understanding the forces at work to keep you balanced in an upright position, just as you learned to walk without first learning the biomechanics involved. Many people are interested in how bicycles work, however. Basically, two forces—*gyroscopic* and *centrifugal*—enable a person to balance on a moving bicycle.

Like a toy gyroscope, a spinning bicycle wheel holds its position in space until upset by an outside force. This force tends to keep a bicycle in balance when in motion.

Centrifugal force is the effect that pushes objects away from the center of a rotating body. You experience this force when you make a sharp curve in a motor vehicle. In bicycle riding, when the cycle starts to fall to one side, correction can be made by turning the bicycle slightly in that direction so that centrifugal force will push you back up again. Keeping balance on a bicycle is largely a series of such corrections. They become so automatic with practice, however, that you do not have to think about them.

A typical bicycle will, for a short distance at least, maintain balance coasting down a hill without a rider. It is also possible to ride a bicycle that is designed so that it will not keep balance when coasting without a rider.

The proper bicycle for learning to ride is not necessarily the right size after the fundamentals have been learned. For learning, or relearning, the saddle should be adjustable and adjusted to the point where the learner can straddle the saddle and easily put both feet flat on the ground outside the pedals. A single-speed bicycle with a coaster brake is generally best. If a geared bicycle is used, place it in one fairly low gear and leave it there. Hand operated brakes tend to make learning more difficult.

Forget about training wheels. It has been my experience that these retard learning, especially for adults. Always wear shoes when you are riding a bicycle, and make sure the bike has a chain guard. A beginner could be seriously injured by catching clothing between the sprocket and chain. Learn in a large open area with a level surface that is hard, smooth, and free of motor vehicle traffic and other obstacles.

To learn or relearn to ride, begin by straddling the saddle. Place your feet on the ground outside the pedals. With the bicycle in a stationary position, practice lifting your feet off the ground. Then place them down again.

Next, learn to move forward by walking your feet along the ground outside the pedals. This is the way *hobby horses* were ridden. Increase your speed slightly and try picking your feet up off the ground and coasting for a short distance before you put your feet down again. Gradually increase the coasting distance with your feet off the ground.

Next, position one pedal forward. This will usually be the right one, but use the left if it feels more natural. Straddle over the saddle. Grip the handlebars, lean forward slightly, and with one foot on the forward pedal, push down on the pedal. Coast. Return your feet to the ground.

Continue to practice in this manner, adding additional pedal revolutions as you gain confidence. To stop, back pedal slowly. When the bicycle is nearly at a standstill, take one foot, usually the left, off the pedal and place it on the ground.

To turn, simply point the front wheel in the direction you wish to go.

After you have mastered the basics, the saddle can be raised for more efficient riding. Do not venture onto streets with automobile traffic until you have thoroughly mastered the basic techniques of riding.

Riding Tips

An accomplished bicycle rider does many things differently than a beginner: there are skills and techniques to learn. With practice, these can become automatic, and you will no longer have to think about them. It's important, however, that you don't allow incorrect techniques to become habits, as habits are extremely difficult to change. Riding is a combination posture, balance, pedaling techniques, gear shifting, braking, and even rhythm and breathing.

The most comfortable posture does not always offer the least wind resistance. You might have to sacrifice some comfort if you want maximum efficiency. Dropped handlebars offer a choice of riding positions. With your hands on the lower handlebars, lean your body well forward. This offers less wind resistance than when you are sitting upright. The leaning forward position might take some getting used to. Sore back and neck muscles might result at first. Alternating leaning forward with a more upright posture is often helpful. Flat handlebars are often preferred by those who lack the fitness or desire to assume an extreme forward leaning position.

The type and height of saddle will also have a bearing on your posture. Perhaps the most comfortable (although this point is often debated), is a very low positioned, padded, mattress-type saddle, which allows the rider to sit nearly upright. This is certainly not the most efficient riding position, however, as far as either wind resistance or pedaling is concerned. Your leg muscles can exert the most power when they can be fully extended, and low saddle height leaves the legs bent even at the low points in the pedal cycles.

A wide saddle interferes with leg motion, especially when the saddle is positioned up high. A narrow saddle allows your thighs to be fairly close together. The saddle can be placed high so that the legs will be almost fully extended when they are on the pedals in the lowest position of the pedal cycle.

When there is no wind, or you are riding into the wind, ride leaning well forward to reduce the resistance as much as possible. When you have a tailwind, however, it is often advantageous to ride in an upright position so that your body acts like a sail.

Many balance factors are more complicated to describe than to execute. Up to a point, balance becomes easier as the speed increases. Using low gears to start out will make balance easier while you are picking up speed.

Beginning riders frequently exhibit considerable side-to-side motion, but experienced riders do not. The difference is just a matter of practice.

Pedaling techniques are important. The use of ankle and foot action can add additional muscle groups to the pedaling. This can be done to a certain extent without toe clips and straps, but the clips and straps greatly increase effectiveness. They also allow you to lift upward on the pedals as well as pushing downward, which is ideal for exercise and physical fitness riding.

Another important factor is the pedaling rate or *cadence*. This is part of the reason why bicycle gears are frequently called *speeds*. In general, bicycle riding at a constant pedaling rate is most efficient. Changing speeds is costly in terms of energy use. Most riders have an optimal rate of pedaling, usually somewhere between 60 and 85 pedal revolutions per minute. At this constant cadence each different gear ratio will give a different speed. Therefore, instead of saying a "10-gear bicycle," the term "10-speed bicycle" is used.

There will, of course, be gear ratios or riding conditions that will not allow the rider to maintain the optimum cadence. Beginners typically use gear ratios that are so high that they cannot possibly keep up their optimal pedaling rate. Stop and start pedaling, in spite of what it might appear, is inefficient. Accelerations require much more effort than maintaining a constant speed.

Experienced riders tend to spend much more time pedaling at their optimum cadence than do beginners. It's extremely difficult to convince a beginner that there is something better than to pedal hard for a short time, coast and rest, and then pedal hard again. For exercise and physical fitness riding, the optimal cadence is most beneficial, at least from an endurance and cardiovascular point of view.

Breathing is closely related to pedaling cadence. Like endurance runners, bicyclists develop rhythmical breathing patterns that coordinate with their leg actions. Except for short sprints, where your breath can be held, breathing should be regular. At least make certain that you do not hold your breath.

Gear Shifting

Gear shifting is extremely important if maximum riding efficiency is to be achieved. The human body operates most efficiently over a narrow range of power output, and the gears allow most effective use of this power. This is why such a large number of gears are frequently used on bicycles. The typical automobile engine can operate effectively over a fairly wide range of power outputs with only three or four gear ratios. A bicycle rider can use 10 or even 15 to advantage.

To correctly shift most internal-hub gears, stop pedaling, shift into another gear while the bicycle is coasting, and then resume pedaling. The actual shifting is done when the chain is *not* moving. Shifting can also be done when at a standstill.

Practice until shifting can be done smoothly and quickly with only a brief pause in the pedaling. Since each gear is in a definite click or notched position, there is generally no problem in finding the gear position.

Derailleur gears require much more skill to operate correctly. The gears are usually shifted by continuous motion of the changer lever without having notches or other set locations for the individual gears. Shifting is largely a matter of feel, and it can take considerable practice to learn this.

The limits can be in set positions as far as the control levers will go either forward or backwards, but even here fine adjustments are usually required to eliminate noise from the derailleur mechanisms.

To shift, ease up on the pedaling, but do not stop completely. Shift by slowly moving the control lever. You should only shift from one sprocket to the next at a time. Avoid skipping sprockets. After shifting, resume normal pedal cadence again. Practice shifting until it can be done smoothly and efficiently.

On five-speed bicycles, there is usually only one control lever, which makes everything easier. There is only one basic pattern to learn. Pull the lever toward you for lower gears and push the lever away from you (releasing tension on the control cable) for higher gears.

On 10-speed and 15-speed bicycles, the operation is complicated somewhat by having two control levers. Regardless of whether the gear control levers are located on the lower frame tube, the handlebar stem, the handlebar tips, or elsewhere, the rear control lever is usually located on the right side of the bicycle. The front derailleur control is on the left side.

On most bicycles, the front derailleur works in the opposite direction of the rear one. Pulling the front derailleur lever toward you shifts into higher gears. On some models, however, the front derailleur works just the opposite. Pulling the lever toward you shifts into lower gears, just like the rear derailleur. I prefer this arrangement.

Do not shift both the front and rear derailleurs at the same time. The key technique is to master a feel for when to shift in order to maintain cadence. In traffic, try to down shift while you are slowing down so that you will be in a low gear when you start out again.

Shifting on hills generally places the greatest stresses on the derailleur mechanisms and the chain. To minimize this, downshift early, before you are struggling to maintain cadence and *lugging* with slow, heavy pedaling.

Many, perhaps most, 10-speed and 15-speed bicycles don't have 10 or 15 effective gear ratios. Some of the ratios are typically so close together, or possibly even the same, as to render them ineffective. It is best to avoid the extreme chain angles, especially from the smallest inside chainwheel to the smallest outside rear sprocket and from the largest outside chainwheel to the largest inside rear sprocket. Try to do most of your riding in gears where the chainwheel and rear sprockets are most nearly lined up. Of course, this will automatically be the case if the gear ratios are properly selected on the bicycle in the first place, and most of your riding will be in the center range of gear values.

Most sprocket arrangements require alternate shifting of the front and rear derailleurs in order to use the full range of gears progressively. After shifting to a new gear, fine adjustments to eliminate noises can be made after pedaling resumes normal cadence. This is a very sensitive adjustment. Move the control lever slightly in one direction until the noise has been eliminated. If it gets worse, move the control lever in the other direction until the noise stops.

Since shifting is largely by feel, you have to get used to each particular bicycle. A switch to another bicycle requires learning another particular method. The adjustment can be even more difficult if the gear ratios are different, the bicycle is lighter or heavier, or the shift control is located in a different place. With enough riding, a particular bicycle becomes like a part of you, and the gear shifting becomes so natural that you don't have to consciously think about it.

Braking

Perhaps the easiest system to operate is the coaster brake. All that is required is simple backward pedaling. There is some skill in applying the required amount of pressure for the particular stopping conditions. The braking should be done smoothly when space and conditions permit, but quickly in certain emergencies.

Bicycles with a single, hand-operated brake to the rear wheel, such as a disk brake, operate similarly to a coaster brake, except that the braking control is by hand. The pedaling, of course, should stop when the braking begins.

Some bicycles have a rear coaster brake and a hand-operated front-wheel brake, usually a caliper brake. In this case, apply the coaster brake first, followed by the hand brake. Never apply the hand brake alone when riding at high speeds, because this can cause the rear wheel to come off the ground, with loss of control and a possible spill the result.

The principles are the same with front and rear hand brakes, except that everything is done by hand. The control handle for the rear brake is generally located on the handlebar on the right side of the bike. The front brake is on the left. The pattern is the same as for derailleur shift levers.

When you are first learning, start to apply the rear brake first, followed by the front brake. Experienced riders apply both brakes at the same time and about equally, but this requires practice.

When coasting downhill, apply the brakes periodically rather than continuously. Don't wait too long before starting the braking. Always keep the speed down to the point where you are well within the capabilities of your braking system.

When riding in traffic, brake *safety levers* (Fig. 8-34) allow you to brake while gripping the upper portion of the handlebars. These add only slightly to the weight of the bicycle.

Cornering

For cornering, try to come into the turn at a slow enough speed so that braking will not be necessary during the turn. If the bicycle has a low bottom bracket in relation to the road level or long cranks, the pedal on the turning side should not be in the down position when making a sharp or high speed turn. Avoid making high speed turns on road surfaces covered with dirt, sand, or gravel, as these conditions can cause sudden side—slippage of one or both wheels.

Safety

Bicycle riding in motor traffic lanes can be dangerous and requires defensive bicycling. If at all possible, do your exercise and physical fitness riding on bicycle paths or where there is no danger from automobiles.

Here are some useful safety rules:

□ Obey traffic rules and signs.
□ Keep your bicycle in good condition. The appearance of the bicycle is secondary to

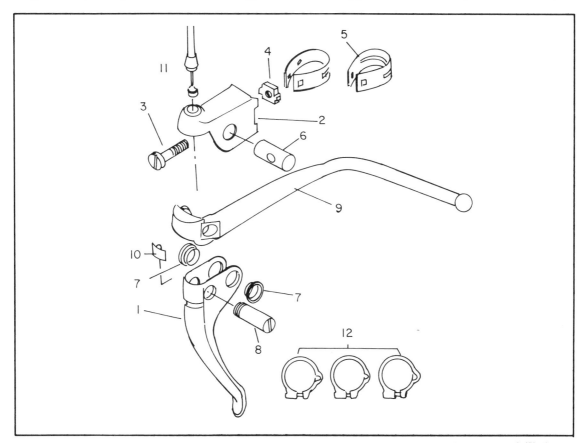

Fig. 8-34. Brake lever with extension lever. Parts are: (1) lever, (2) lever bracket, (3) pull-up bolt, (4) pull-up nut, (5) clamp, (6) pull-up stud, (7) flanged thrust washer, (8) cable anchor stud, (9) extension lever, (10) extension lever spring, (11) cable set, and (12) outer band for frame tube.

mechanical condition when it comes to safety. Faulty brakes are a common cause of accidents.

□ Use safety equipment such as reflectors and lights for night riding. These safety accessories might be required by law in the area where you are bicycling. Even if they are not, you should have equipment that will add to the safety of the riding you do.

□ Whenever possible, use bikeways, bicycle paths, and trails. There is a growing network of these in the United States. Not only is it safer, but also a much more pleasurable experience to be able to ride completely free of worry about automobile traffic.

□ Develop safe and sensible habits. Watch the road for potholes, cracks, drain covers, and rail tracks. Be especially careful in wet conditions. If caliper brakes become wet, dry them out by riding with light applications of the brakes so that they will be ready when you need them. Certain weather and traffic conditions make it unsafe to bicycle, especially at night.

□ Always be alert for such things as car doors opening and cars parking or pulling out.

□ Yield the right-of-way and show respect for pedestrians. Do this even though motorists may not give you the same courtesy.

Helmets and Head Gear

Helmets and head gear are important safety accessories. Many newer helmets provide considerable protection while still being lightweight and comfortable to wear. I recommend helmets not only for racing, where they are standard equipment, but also for exercise and physical fitness riding.

Legal Requirements

Legal requirements vary across the country. Find out what they are for the area where you will be riding your bicycle. City, county, or state registration might be required in addition to certain safety equipment. Most bicycle dealers can give you accurate information about the legal requirements for a particular area. Be sure to record the serial number of your bicycle and register it if required in the area where you live.

Transporting Bicycles

In some cases, you will need to transport your bicycle by automobile to a safe area for exercise and physical fitness riding. A number of racks are available for transporting bicycles on automobiles. The three basic types are rear bumper racks, roof racks, and rear deck racks.

Features to look for in racks are the number of bicycles that can be transported, ease of getting bicycles on and off the racks, secure methods of attaching racks to vehicles and bicycles to the racks, and protection of vehicles and bicycles from damage.

TOOLS FOR MAINTENANCE AND REPAIRS

You can generally save money in the long run by purchasing top quality tools made of heat treated alloy steel. For best results, keep tools clean and organized. After using a tool, wipe off dirt and grease with a cloth. Keep tools together in a toolbox or on a pegboard rack or some other special place. Keep sets of wrenches together. Avoid using tools for purposes other than those for which they were designed. Time spent keeping tools clean and in order will usually save time in making repairs.

For most routine bicycle servicing and maintenance only a few tools are essential, but these will need to be selected carefully. Not having the right tool for the particular job is one of the greatest pitfalls in mechanics. Pliers, for example, make very poor substitutes for wrenches and almost the right size wrench is not the same thing as having the right size. It is frustrating to start a job and get part way through it, only to find that you don't have an essential tool to complete the work.

While regular mechanics tools will suffice for many jobs, you will probably want to have at least a few tools designed specifically for bicycle use.

Useful standard tools include crescent wrenches, pliers, screwdrivers, cable cutters, open-end and box wrenches, socket wrenches, and Allen wrenches. A number of special bicycle wrenches may be useful. Special flat bicycle wrenches, commonly called *cone wrenches*, are extra thin, open-ended wrenches. As the name implies, they are designed especially for use on hub cones and lock nuts. They are available in both American Standard and metric sizes. There are also special wrenches for caliper hand brakes, derailleurs, etc. Special bicycle wrenches with a number of open-end and box openings in the same tool are especially handy for carrying in bicycle repair kits. A typical wrench will fit the pedals, cones, locknuts, saddle and handlebar clamps, and brake-shoe pad nuts.

Spoke wrenches are used for tightening and loosening spokes. They can be purchased at bicycle shops, and are needed for trueing wheels, replacing broken spokes, lacing wheels, and similar jobs. There are several sizes, so make certain that you get the size that fits the spokes on the wheels you intend to work on.

Tire levers are useful for changing bicycle tires. They are available in small sizes designed especially for bicycles. Those with notches that fit over spokes and hold the tire bead off the rim are especially handy.

Chain tools are used to remove rivets from chains. They are required for taking derailleur chains apart.

There are a number of other special tools that are either essential for doing certain jobs or else make the work easier or faster. For example, there are tools for removing freewheels from the hubs, brake arm clamping tools called "third-hands," and tools for removing cotters from pedal arms. These and other special tools and their uses are detailed later in this chapter.

While it might seem like there are an endless number of bicycle tools, only a few tools are required to disassemble and assemble everything on a particular bicycle. Of course, they must be the right tools and sizes.

Other useful tools include hammers, files, hacksaws, drills, screw extractors, center punches, and dies and taps. Dies and taps, for example, are handy for cleaning up damaged threads on bolts and nuts. A drill and tap extractor can be used to remove broken bolts by drilling a hole in the center of the broken bolt.

The extractor is tapped into the hole with a hammer, and a wrench is used to turn the extractor for removing the broken bolt.

For bicycle repair work, as well as most other types of shop work, a sturdy workbench with a mounted heavy-duty vise is extremely useful.

Maintenance Stands and Cleaning Supplies

Maintenance stands, also called repair racks and tune-up stands, are used to hold bicycles firmly off the ground so that repairs and adjustments can be made. They allow you to work the pedals by hand and operate the shift and brake controls. Many of these racks allow you to position the bicycle almost any way you want it for a particular job you are doing, such as right side up, upside down, or at any desired angle. Basically, the rack holds the bicycle so that your hands are free to do other things.

You can, of course, get along without a rack by simply turning the bicycle upside down and balancing it on the saddle and handlebars. The bicycle may lack stability in this position, however, be too low for convenient work, and possibly be damaging to the bicycle.

Maintenance racks are useful devices not only for bicycle builders and mechanics, but also for the one-bicycle owner. The racks are available in self-supporting models and for attachment to floors and walls in a range of prices.

Cleaning parts is an important part of bicycle mechanics. Cleaning pans can be purchased from automobile supply stores. You can also use any suitable container that will withstand the solvents that you intend to use.

Kerosene works well as a cleaning solvent for bicycle parts. Special solvents that work similarly are also available. Kerosene and other solvents are available from automotive stores and service stations. *Do not use gasoline as a cleaning solvent.*

You will need a supply of rags, cleaner, polish, and wax suitable for the finishes on your bicycle. You will also need grease and oil lubricants, as detailed later in this chapter.

It is usually easiest to replace parts with the same brands and models as were used previously. If these are not available, it is often possible to substitute other brands.

In many cases, if one part of a component is damaged, it works best to replace the entire unit, especially in the case of inexpensive components. On more expensive components, it is sometimes worth the trouble to replace only the part that is causing the difficulty.

A number of universal replacement parts, such as caliper brakes and shift changers, can be useful. "Universal," in this context, usually means that they will fit several or most brands of bicycles that use similar components.

In most cases, you will probably want to use new parts when making replacements, but there are times when used parts will serve your purposes just about as well and save you money.

Many bicycle dealers have large stocks of bicycle parts. Another possibility is to order them by mail. Mail order companies include:

—Big-Wheel Ltd., 340 Holly Street, Denver, CO 80221.

—Cycl-Ology, Wheel Goods Corporation, 14524 21st Avenue North, Minneapolis, MN 55441.

—Cyclo-Pedia, 311 N. Mitchell, Cadillac, MI 49601.

MAINTENANCE AND REPAIRS

Some basic lubricating tasks require that you disassemble parts, clean them, apply lubrication, and then reassemble them. This is commonly called an "overhaul." The first time that you do this will usually be the most difficult. After a few times it will probably become routine.

Some bicycles come with maintenance manuals complete with schematics. These can be a big help. If you don't have a manual for your particular bicycle, try to get one from the manufacturer. To learn the workings of a particular bicycle, study the bike as you read about it. It helps to have the bicycle in a maintenance rack.

Before starting any job, make certain you have all the tools and supplies you will need and that spare parts are available.

The most common types of fasteners used to connect bicycle components are nuts and machine screws or bolts. In order to join a nut and bolt, both the diameters and thread patterns must match. When the threads are in good condition, the match up can be tested by turning

the nut on the bolt by hand. If this cannot be done and the thread are not damaged, you probably do not have a matched set.

Machine screws have various head types, including hex, flat, oval, and round with either slotted, Phillips, or Allen openings. The most common nuts used on bikes are ordinary nuts, self-locking nuts, and wing nuts. Two types of washers—flat and lock—are commonly used.

When making fastener replacements, it is a good idea to take the damaged or broken ones with you to the hardware store or bicycle shop so that you can get exact matchups. While substitutes can sometimes be used, it's generally best to stick with the same size and type as the original.

Maintenance Schedules

Maintenance should be kept in perspective. If you are mainly interested in using your bicycle for exercise and physical fitness riding, then you may only want to do the minimum maintenance work necessary to keep your bicycle in safe operating condition. You will probably also want the bicycle to perform well.

Considering the relatively low cost of the investment, don't make yourself a slave to a maintenance program unless you enjoy it. You should do at least enough maintenance, or have it done for you, to keep the bicycle in safe operating condition.

Keeping a bicycle stored out of the weather, dry, waxed, and properly lubricated will help keep it in top condition, but there are many happy bicycle riders on "rusty wonders," too.

Lubrication is a primary concern if you want to keep a bicycle in top operating condition and precision. Follow the instructions that come with the particular bicycle for the proper procedure.

In general, front hubs with oil fittings should have about a ½ teaspoonful of light bicycle oil added about once a month. Most front bicycle hubs to not have oil fittings and are lubricated with grease rather than oil. Do not apply oil to these, as this will only wash away the grease.

Coaster-brake rear hubs are lubricated in various ways, depending on the particular assembly. On hubs with oil fittings, a ½ teaspoonful of light bicycle oil is usually recommended about once a month. Many coaster brake hubs are lubricated with both grease and oil, and some require disassembly for complete lubrication. Follow the manufacturer's instructions.

Internal-geared hubs usually have oil fittings. Oil is added as described above for coaster brake hubs with oil fittings, except that more oil is required for the internal-geared hubs. Follow the manufacturer's recommendations.

For freewheels, add a few drops of light oil to the freewheel mechanism about once a month. This is done externally. For maximum performance, the freewheel should be removed from the bicycle (but not disassembled), cleaned, and oiled about every six months.

For derailleur mechanisms, add light oil to the pivot points on front and rear derailleur mechanisms and to the jockey and tension wheels on the rear derailleur. Apply oil sparingly to control levers, but avoid getting oil on the friction surfaces that keep the controls from slipping positions.

Chains should ideally be removed monthly, cleaned in kerosene or other suitable solvent, lubricated with bicycle chain oil, and reinstalled. If this schedule is too severe, simply wipe the chain with a cloth, add bicycle chain oil sparingly, and wipe excess off. The removal, cleaning, and relubricating can be done every six months. Chain maintenance is especially important on derailleur bicycles, because shifting and chain angles place considerable stresses on the chain.

Conventional pedals often have a small hole for adding a few drops of bicycle oil about once a month. Some conventional pedals and most rattraps should be overhauled with grease about every six months. Do not add oil to these.

Add a few drops of bicycle oil to the brake and gear change cables where they enter housings about once a month.

Add bicycle oil to the pivot points of brake calipers about once a month. Avoid getting oil on the rubber brake pads.

You should routinely check that all nuts and bolts are properly tightened. Multi-speed hubs, derailleurs, and caliper brakes should be adjusted whenever they are not working properly. Inspections should be made at monthly intervals.

Frequent wiping of dust, dirt, and road soil from the bicycle frame and components will help to keep the bicycle in top condition. Some people wash bicycles with soap and water, but I do not think much of this idea, because water is likely to enter the internal workings and wash away lubricants. If you do use this method, dry the bicycle off as thoroughly as possible afterwards.

Cleaning compounds, polishes, and waxes can be used on painted, plated, and metal surfaces, but take special care here, as many products can be more harmful than beneficial. Avoid especially harsh and abrasive compounds. Waxes that are specially compounded for bicycles are available at bicycle shops, some in spray cans. Because of the high risk of breathing harmful chemicals, however, I do not recommend these. Instead, purchase the less expensive waxes in liquid or paste form and apply them with a cloth.

In addition, front hubs, head sets, and pedals should be taken apart, cleaned, lubricated, and reassembled about every six months if they are to be maintained in top working precision. Rear hubs and crank sets should be overhauled about once a year.

The basic procedure is to mount the bicycle in a maintenance rack and service one assembly at a time. You might want to start with the front hub. Remove the front wheel. Disassemble the hub. Clean all parts in kerosene or other suitable solvent. A pan or bowl partly filled with cleaning fluid can be positioned under the part to be cleaned. For parts that cannot be submerged in the cleaning fluid, apply with a brush. Even if you have a big enough pan and enough cleaning fluid, don't submerge the tire and tube to clean the center hub.

After thoroughly cleaning the parts by soaking and/or brushing the solvent on them, allow the fluid to completely dry or evaporate. Wipe with a cloth to make certain that no cleaning fluid remains. Check the condition of all components and make replacements as required.

Add lubrication to the bearings. In the case of loose bearings (those not contained in a retainer), the individual balls can be held in position with grease while the assembly is being made. Reassemble the hub and install the wheel

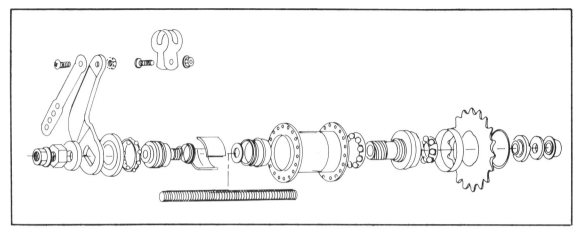

Fig. 8-35. Coaster brake hub assembly.

back on the bicycle. Then go on to another component.

Unless you have fairly advanced mechanical skills, I do not recommend taking coaster brake (Fig. 8-35) and internal gear hubs (Fig. 8-36) apart. They are fairly complicated as bicycle assemblies go and generally have a long life expectancy without overhauls. If internal repairs are required, you may want to have this work done at a bicycle shop for a number of reasons. There are a multitude of different hubs in use, making the likelihood of finding parts for a particular hub questionable. It is often difficult for an amateur mechanic to determine the specific problem: the hub might not even be worth repairing, because the replacement parts could cost more than an entire new hub. The time required for the amateur to do the job can be considerable and possibly not worth the trouble. Special tools may be required. For routine servicing when no repairs are needed, the advantages gained by overhauling coaster brake hubs is probably not worth the risks.

If you do want to tackle these jobs, try to get the assembly drawings for the particular hub from the manufacturer. If you can't get the drawings, take special care to note the order that the pieces come apart so that you will be able to reassemble them again. It might be helpful to make diagrams.

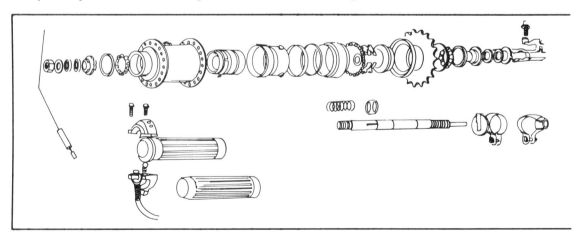

Fig. 8-36. Internal gear hub assembly.

Tires and Tubes

Tires and tubes are a vulnerable part of a bicycle. Even if precautions are taken to prevent punctures or other damage while riding, the tires will sooner or later wear out. The quality and type of tires selected plays an important part in their useful life.

Keeping a tire inflated at proper pressure is important and should become a part of routine maintenance. Under- or over-inflation can make riding more difficult and less comfortable, and both of these conditions can lead to tire and tube damage.

Changing tires and tubes and patching tubes are relatively simple repair tasks. These jobs are fairly costly when you have them done at bicycle shops.

Maintaining proper tire inflation is extremely important. The tubes used with clincher tires generally have *Schraeder* valves, while tubular tubes use the *Presta* valve. These require different air hose attachments to fit them. There is an inexpensive adapter, however, that allows Presta valves to be filled with the Schraeder air hose fittings. The Schraeder valves can be inflated with the conventional pumps found at gas stations. Hand pumps are available for either type of tube valves.

It can be risky to attempt to inflate tires at filling stations. The air pressure available is usually much greater than is needed and this makes blowouts easily possible. A hand bicycle pump with a built-in gauge is a much better method. Make certain the pump you select is easy to work and efficient. Inflating a tire is almost impossible with some of the cheaper hand pumps that are on the market. If the pump does not have a built-in gauge, use a high-pressure tire gauge. These can be purchased at bicycle shops and automotive stores.

Due to the porosity of materials, it's normal for tubes to lose air over a period of time. The proper tire pressure, usually given as a range of pressures, is typically shown on the side of the tire.

If the valve stem does not extend straight through the hole in the rim on an inflated tube, remove some of the air by depressing or loosening the valve in the stem. Rotate the tube inside the tire until the valve is straight in the rim hole. Then reinflate.

A common problem when inflating a tire is improper seating of the tire on the rim. To avoid this, partially inflate the tire. Check seating and alignment. Make necessary corrections with your hands. Then inflate to desired pressure. If seating or alignment is still incorrect, partially deflate and try again.

You will need a tube repair kit for repairing small holes in clincher tubes. These can be purchased at bicycle shops and auto stores.

To make changes or repairs on clinchers, first remove the wheel from the bicycle. With a tire lever (the type with a notch to hook over a spoke is recommended) lift one bead of the tire over the edge of the rim. Take care not to pinch the tube or stretch the wire bead any more than is absolutely necessary. Hook the tire lever to a spoke. If you have the type of tire lever without a spoke notch, hold it back by hand. The difficulty, of course, is in having enough hands—one reason for the spoke notches.

With a second tire lever about 4 inches from the first one, lift the tire bead over the rim and lock the tire lever to a spoke. If necessary, use a third tire lever about 4 inches from one of the others. Free the tire bead on one side of the tire from the rim all the way around. On tubes with a nut holding the valve to the rim, remove the nut. Remove the tube from the rim.

Always thoroughly check the tire both inside and out to make certain that whatever caused the puncture is not still present. Inflate the tube. If it is important to make repairs quickly, try to locate punctures by inspection. If holes cannot be located in this manner, place the inflated tube in a basin or pan of water and watch for air bubbles. Mark holes with chalk. If the water test was used, a tube must be allowed to dry thoroughly before patching.

To patch a tube, clean and roughen area where the patch is to be applied. Roughen around the hole with sandpaper or use the rasp-holes on the lid of the patching kit container. Do this carefully: if poorly done, leaking around the patch will be likely. Spread an even layer of patching adhesive over the roughened area and allow it to thoroughly dry. While waiting, you can trim the corners of a patch if they are not already rounded. Sharp corners tend to work loose. The adhesive should be dry before backing is removed from the patch. When removing the backing, take care not to touch the surface of the patch. Apply the patch, working it in place and stretching it to the tube. If the tube is replaced right away, sprinkle talcum powder around the area of the patch to help prevent sticking.

If a hole in the tube is on the rim side, examine the inside of the rim. One common cause is for a spoke that has been tightened too for to protrude past the nipple. It will punch through the rim liner and puncture the tube.

Deflate the tube. Insert the valve stem in the hole in the rim first. Then work the tube inside the tire all the way around. Smooth the tube so that there are no twists. Push the tire bead back over the rim with your thumbs. Inflate the tire to proper pressure. Make sure that the tire is properly seated and the valve stem is straight. If not, deflate, make adjustments, and reinflate. If there is a valve stem nut, thread in place and tighten down. Always use a valve cap to keep dirt out of the valve.

The procedure for replacing a tire is the same except that the second bead is also removed from the rim on the same side of the rim as the first bead was removed. Do this by hand.

Tubular repairs generally take much longer than clinchers. To avoid delays, touring cyclists who use tubulars often carry extra tires with the tubes already sewn in place. These fold up and are easy to carry. When on the road, a flat tire is removed and replaced with one of these spares.

To make tubular repairs, you will need patches that are usually thinner than those used for clinchers and adhesive, curved needle, linen thread, rim cement, roughening lid that is often found on patching kit containers or sandpaper, razor blade or stitch cutters, talcum powder, and chalk.

To remove a tire, first break loose the cement holding the tire to the rim. No tire irons are required. Start near the valve stem. Using both thumbs, roll the tire off the rim. Work progressively around the rim.

Try to locate the leak before removing the tube from the tire. This will make it possible to repair the hole while removing a minimum of stitching. Restitching is a time consuming job, so it's important to keep it to a minimum. Sometimes the leak can be located by finding the object that caused it. If you can't find the hole in this manner, pump some air into the tube and listen for the leak. If you still can't locate it, submerge both the tire and tube together.

After the leak has been located, mark with chalk. Strip back the tape that covers the stitches in that area. A couple of inches of working space is usually ample. Using a razor blade or stitch cutting tool, remove about 1½-inch of the stitches.

Remove a section of the tube through the opening in the tire and locate the hole in the tube. Follow procedures given above for patching clincher tubes, except use a special, thinner patch that is designed for sew-ups.

Work the tube back inside the tire. Use needle and thread to resew the tire. Space stitches about ⅜-inch apart. Cement tape back over stitches with rim cement.

Apply cement to the rim, not to the tire. Old cement need not be removed. Wait until cement becomes tacky—usually only a few minutes—then mount the tire. Start with the valve stem and work the tire on around the rim in both directions from the valve stem. When the tire is on the rim all the way around, rotate the tire until it is centered. This must be done quickly while the cement is still tacky. An even amount of sidewall should show all the way around on both sides of the tire.

Inflate the tire. Allow time for the cement to set before riding. If you must ride immediately, ride slowly, and avoid turns that could work the tire off the rim.

Hubs and Freewheels

Figure 8-37 shows a typical hub and bearing arrangement with axle nuts. A quick-release hub is shown in Fig. 8-38. Both hubs shown use the same basic bearing arrangement, used on almost all front and rear hubs, including those with internal gears and coaster brakes. In essence, the only links between the hub shell and the axle are the bearings.

A new design uses permanently sealed bearings, which can go for long periods of time

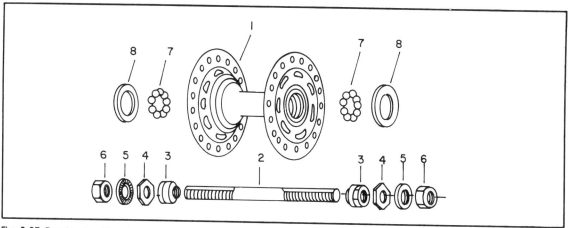

Fig. 8-37. Front hub with axle nuts. Parts are: (1) hub shell, (2) axle, (3) cone, (4) lock nut, (5) washer, (6) axle nut, (7) steel ball, (8) dust cap, and (9) axle set.

without maintenance. When the bearings finally do wear out, the sealed bearing units are usually replaced with new ones.

A frequent cause of excessive wheel play between the axle and hub is loose cones. In turn, wheels that will not spin freely frequently have cones that are too tight. Simple adjustments will correct these problems. Of course, the problem might also be something more serious, such as lack of lubrication or worn parts, but always check the cone adjustment first.

The cones on some inexpensive bicycles do not have lock nuts. Instead, the cones are locked in place by the axle nut when the axle is installed on a bicycle frame. This is a poor arrangement, as it is difficult to remove the wheel without losing the cone adjustment. A simple improvement is to add thin lock nuts. There is usually ample space to fit these in.

To adjust cones without lock nuts, loosen one of the axle mounting nuts. It isn't necessary to remove the wheel from the bicycle. Using a

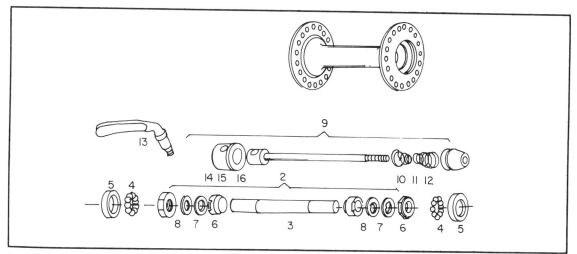

Fig. 8-38. Front hub with quick release. Parts are: (1) hub shell, (2) complete axle set, (3) axle, (4) bearings, (5) dust cap, (6) cone, (7) key washer, (8) lock nut, (9) complete quick release unit, (10) skewer, (11) volute spring, (12) nut for skewer, (13) cam lever, (14) body cam lever, and (15) cap nut.

wrench that fits the cone, loosen the cone, then tighten until the bearings are seated firmly. This pulls the two cones closer together so both bearings are affected equally. Do not over-tighten, since this can cause damage. Next, loosen the cone approximately a half turn. Hold the cone in this position with a wrench and tighten the axle nut with another wrench.

The wheel should now turn freely without excessive play. If not, try to make further fine adjustments. Loosen the cone another quarter turn if the wheel does not turn freely. If the wheel has excessive play, tighten the cone a quarter turn. If several such adjustments do not correct the problem, it probably means lack of lubrica-tion or worn or damaged parts inside the hub. You will need to disassemble the hub to find and correct the problem.

To adjust cones with lock nuts, loosen one of the axle mounting nuts. It isn't necessary to remove the wheel from the bicycle. You will need a thin wrench that fits the cone and another thin wrench that fits the lock nut. Hold the cone with one wrench and loosen the lock nut with the other wrench. Tighten the cone until the bearings are firmly seated. Take care not to over-tighten. Loosen the cone a half turn; hold the cone in this position with one wrench and tighten the lock nut against the cone with the second wrench. Retighten the axle nut. The wheel should now turn freely without excessive play. If not, make fine adjustments as described above for cones without lock nuts. If this does not cure the problem, you will need to overhaul the hub.

To adjust the cones on a quick-release hub, open the quick release lever and remove the wheel from the bicycle. Adjust one cone as detailed above for cones with lock nuts. Rein-stall the wheel on the bicycle.

To overhaul a hub, you will need to remove the wheel from the bicycle, disassemble the hub center, clean, inspect, and replace parts as re-quired, lubricate, reassemble, and reinstall the wheel on the bicycle.

This work is best done with the bicycle in a repair rack. The following basic steps, with noted differences, apply to most standard front and rear hubs without internal gears or brakes, including those with fixed and freewheel sprockets.

Begin the overhaul by removing the wheel from the bicycle. If you are going to overhaul both the front and rear hubs, it is generally best to do one at a time. Finish one wheel and reinstall it before starting the second wheel.

Hub assemblies are shown in Figs. 8-39 and Fig. 8-40. Even though the rear hubs have sprockets, with or without free-wheeling, the axle and bearing assemblies are basically the same as for the front hubs.

Begin disassembly by removing axle mounting nuts or quick release assembly. The quick release assembly is removed by holding the cam lever and unscrewing the nut for the skewer, removing the tension or volute spring, and sliding the skewer out of the axle center. The remainder of the quick release need not be disassembled unless parts such as the cam lever are to be replaced.

For hubs with freewheels, the next step is to remove the freewheel (Fig. 8-41). There are two special types of removal tools: for freewheels with splines and for freewheels with lugs. Make sure that you get the right one for your free-wheel. You will also need a vise with copper jaws or a special device that goes in a vise for holding threaded axles.

Mount the axle in the copper jaws of the vice or in the special axle device. Use a wrench to remove the spacer nut from the axle. Some hubs have a lock nut and a spacer: in this case, the lock nut is removed first, then the spacer.

Next, remove the axle and wheel from the vise. Clamp the freewheel removal tool in the vise with the splines or lugs facing upward. With sprockets downward, slip the freewheel over the removal tool. With the tool seated and aligned, rotate the wheel counterclockwise until the hub comes off the freewheel. In some cases, especially with the lug-type of freewheels, it might be necessary to hold the removal tool in position by using an axle nut or reinstalling the quick release assembly. This is only necessary to free the thread hold initially. Once the freewheel is started, remove the nut or quick release assembly and turn the freewheel to remove it from the hub.

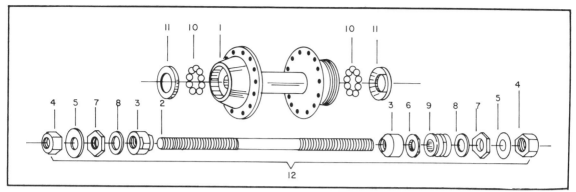

Fig. 8-39. Rear hub assembly with axle nuts. Parts are: (1) hub shell, (2) axle, (3) cone, (4) axle nut, (5) lock washer, (6) lock nut, (7) lock nut, (8) spacer, (9) spacer, (10) steel ball, (11) dust cap, and (12) axle set.

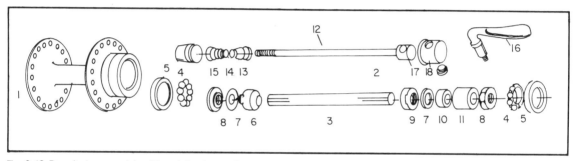

Fig. 8-40. Rear hub assembly with quick release. Parts are: (1) hub shell, (2) complete axle set, (3) axle, (4) steel ball, (5) dust cap, (6) cone, (7) key washer, (8) lock nut, (9) cone, (10) lock nut, (11) spacer, (12) complete quick release unit, (13) skewer, (14) volute spring, (15) nut for skewer, (16) cam lever, (17) body cam lever, and (18) cap nut.

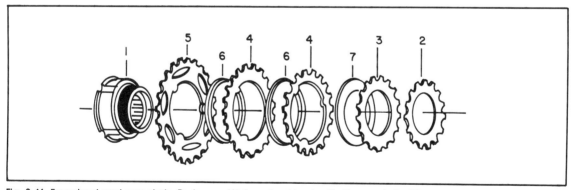

Fig. 8-41. Freewheel and sprockets. Parts are: (1) freewheel body, (2-5) sprockets, (6) spacer A, and (7) spacer B.

I do not recommend that you try to disassemble the freewheel unit itself. Special tools are required for removing the sprockets from the freewheel. If you need to remove these to make a switch or replacement, I suggest that you take the unit to a bicycle shop and have the job done for you. For cleaning, soak the freewheel and sprockets as a unit in solvent. Drain, allow to dry, and wipe with cloth. A brush can be used with the solvent to clean between the sprockets.

207

When the unit is completely clean and dry, oil the freewheel with light bicycle oil. The unit is then ready for reassembly to the hub.

For regular hub overhaul, you won't need to remove the spoke protector. For some jobs, such as wheel spoking, this will be necessary. Some hubs also have a spacer washer between the spoke protector and hub.

Next, clamp the lock nut on one end of the axle in a vise or hold it with a wrench on the downward side of the hub. If the hub has no lock nut, form one by tightening an axle nut against the cone. With an appropriate wrench, loosen and remove the lock nut on the upward end of the axle, if present. Then remove the cone and slide the axle out of the hub.

There are two basic types of bearing arrangements: bearings caged in retainers and loose bearings. Those in retainers can be removed as a unit. The loose kind are covered by dust caps. The balls can be removed individually. Tweezers can be used for picking out the individual balls. It's a good idea to count them so that you will know how many go back. Next, turn the hub over and remove the bearings from the other end.

The remaining cone on the axle need not be removed unless replacement is necessary. Before removing this cone, first measure the distance of the cone from the end of the axle so you will know where to position it for reassembly.

Clean all parts in solvent, check, and make replacements as necessary. If any of the bearings are worn or pitted, it's best to replace the complete set. Check axle, nuts, and cones for thread damage, and make certain that the axle is not bent.

Reassemble hub in reverse order of disassembly, except that bearings are packed in bicycle grease. The grease will also serve to hold individual loose bearings in position until assembly is completed.

After assembly, adjust the cones as detailed above. Hold cone in position with a thin wrench and tighten the lock nut. On hubs where a freewheel was removed, reinstall the freewheel. On quick release hubs, install assemblies through axle centers. Put the wheel back on the bicycle.

Coaster-brake and internal-gear hubs will usually give long service without overhaul. If the hub has a grease fitting or oil cap, periodically adding lubrication is all that is normally required. If the hub requires repair, it is usually best done at a bicycle shop, because there are many different models and repairing them can be difficult.

Wheel Trueing

To form a wheel, the rim is connected to the hub flanges by adjustable spokes. Clinchers have a deep U-shaped channel for clincher tires, and tubulars have a slight depression for cementing on sew-up tires. When the spokes are properly adjusted, the wheel will be true and turn smoothly without wobble or up-and-down motion.

Minor adjustments can sometimes be made without removing the wheel from the bicycle and with the tire and tube left in place. There is some risk of puncturing the tube by tightening a spoke nipple to the point where the end of the spoke will extend through the nipple and puncture the tube. (A spoke nipple has internal threads that pass through the rim and holds the spoke in place.) Because most spoked wheels only have the nipple threaded part way over the threaded end of the spoke, however, the risk is only slight that minor tightening will cause a spoke to pass through the nipple. Otherwise, the wheel will have to be removed from the bicycle and the tire, tube, and rim liner removed before the alignment is made.

To true a wheel without removing the wheel from the bicycle or the tire and tube, turn the bicycle upside down or mount it in a maintenance rack so that the wheel can be turned. Using the brake pads or the eraser end of a pencil as a guide, figure out where the wheel is out of alignment. Determine which spokes need to be adjusted. Use a spoke wrench to make the necessary adjustments to the spoke nipples. In many cases, only small adjustments will be required. If the rim is off to one side and too close to the center of the wheel in the same area, the required correction is to loosen the spoke or spokes that are pulling the rim to that side and toward the axle. Try a quarter turn of the spoke or spokes. Then spin the wheel again and check for trueness. Repeat this method until the rim is true.

One or two broken spokes can sometimes be replaced without removing the wheel from the bicycle or the tire and tube from the wheel. The wheel will have to be in near alignment and the spoke or spokes broken in such a way that you can unthread the broken part out of the nipple. If not, you may still be able to make the replacement without removing the wheel from the bicycle by letting the air out of the tire and working the tire and tube to one side where the nipple or nipples are to be replaced. Lift back the rim liner and remove the nipple or nipples. It is best to use exact replacements for both nipples and spokes. Take the broken pieces to a bicycle shop as a guide. In some cases, the sprocket placement will not allow you to insert a spoke in the normal manner. In this case, an extra long spoke can be bent to the correct length. Cut off about ⅜-inch past the bend, insert, and loop in the hub spoke hole. With one or more new spokes in place, tighten the nipple or nipples until they are approximately the same tightness as neighboring spokes. Final adjustments can be made after the tire has been inflated.

If the wheel is too far out of alignment or has too many broken spokes for making corrections as detailed above, major wheel trueing will be required. Since this job requires considerable skill, you may want to take the wheel to a bicycle shop and have this work done for you. If so, it will usually cost you less if you remove the wheel from the bicycle and remove the tire, tube and rim liner from the wheel.

Or you might want to tackle the job yourself. For high performance bicycling, a wheel trueing stand will be needed. These hold the wheel by the axle and have gauges for measuring the trueness of the rim when it rotates. For less precise work, you can improvise a stand by mounting by its stem a bicycle fork turned upside down in a vise. For rear wheels, the axle notches in the fork blades or dropouts can be widened to take the larger axles. The wheel with tire, tube, and rim liner removed is mounted so it can be rotated freely. Fasten a cardboard or tape guide across the fork blades just below the rim, and make a mark in the exact center. Mark half the rim width to each side of the center mark.

Before doing this, however, make certain that the axle of the wheel is exactly perpendicular in the fork prongs.

Front hubs and some non-derailleur rear hubs have the hub centered with the rim. Derailleur hubs are set off to one side of the rim to make room for the wide cluster of sprockets. The rim must be centered between the dropouts so that it will line up exactly with the front wheel and the centerline of the bicycle. To achieve this, different spoke lengths are used on opposite sides of the hub flange. It's called *dishing*.

The improvised truing stand will allow you to center the rim to a fair degree of accuracy. If greater accuracy is required, a trueing gauge or professional trueing stand with precision centering gauge is needed.

A trueing stand, in addition to centering the rim, is used to determine the degree to which the wheel is round and its side-to-side trueness. Deviations can be located and corrections made by tightening and loosening spokes.

Before starting the alignment of a previously used wheel, replace all broken or damaged spokes. Tighten them approximately the same amount as neighboring spokes. The instructions that follow also apply to newly laced wheels.

A wheel with a flattened spot in one area and a bulge in another is corrected by loosening the spokes in the flattened area and tightening the spokes in the bulged area. The areas requiring corrections can be determined by spinning the wheel and watching the guide. Flattened spots are areas where the rim moves away from the guide, closer to the center of the wheel. Bulges are areas where the rim moves closer to the guide, away from the center of the wheel. When the wheel is concentric or exactly round, the rim will remain an equal distance from the guide.

Adjustments in lateral trueness are done last. These generally have little or no effect on roundness. For example, on a 27-inch wheel, the tightening of a spoke one turn and the loosening of the next spoke one full turn will shift the rim about ⅛-inch to the side where the spoke was tightened, while causing very little change in the concentricity.

There is little point in loosening a spoke that is already too loose. A wheel laced by the procedure given later in this chapter should result in approximately the right spoke tensions. If you feel that the spokes are too loose, go around the wheel and tighten each one an additional quarter turn. If they are too tight, loosen each a quarter turn.

Continue making adjustments until you are satisfied with the lateral trueness of the wheel. Correct the major deviations first, before taking care of the minor ones. Make a final check of the concentricity. If this still looks okay, the trueing is completed.

If there are any sharp bends in the rim, you will probably have to replace the rim. In some cases, minor corrections can be made, especially in steel rims, which are usually easier to straighten than alloy rims.

Before putting a rim liner over a clincher rim or cementing on a sew-up tire to a tubular rim, check to make certain that no spokes extend beyond the nipples on the tire side of the rim. If any do, file them off until they are flush with the nipple and smooth. Also, check to make certain that all nipples are properly seated.

Wheel Lacing

Wheel lacing is spoking a rim to a hub. It is actually quite easy once you get the knack of it, but it does take some practice to learn the techniques. Unless you plan to do a number of wheels, you might want to have this work done at a bicycle shop.

A good way to learn wheel lacing is to get an old spoked wheel and use it like a puzzle. Take it apart and put it back together again. Use a freeing oil to help free the nipples from the spoke threads the first time you take the wheel apart. The wheel can also be used to practice wheel trueing.

For an actual lacing job, you will need the correct length and size of spokes. If the rim and hub were previously spoked together, use an old spoke as a pattern. Take it to a bicycle shop with you when buying new spokes. Most bicycle shops also have charts that give spoke lengths and cross patterns for various hubs and rims. Cross patterns refer to the specific number of head-down spokes that each head-up spoke

crosses over. The most common cross patterns are three and four.

On some wheels, especially those used on derailleur bicycles, the spokes will be interlaced. This means that the head up spoke crosses over all but the last of the spokes in the cross pattern and crosses under the last one. This gives added strength and stiffness to the wheel.

The hub will generally have the same number of spoke holes as the rim. This will vary from about 36 to 40 on most 27-inch bicycles.

As a general rule, high quality spokes are the most economical in the long run. I suggest that you do not mix brands on the same wheel. Not all nipples fit all spokes, so make certain you purchase those that do.

When you have the hub, rim, correct length of spokes, and nipples, you are ready to lace the wheel. The holes in most rims are drilled off-center. Every other hole is off to one side of the rim. The holes on opposite flanges of the hub are not directly across from each other, but staggered. A hole on the flange on one side will line up exactly midway between two holes on the opposite flange.

Some hubs have countersunk holes. These are not to set the spoke heads flush, but rather to reduce the stress from the sharp bends in the spokes. The spoke head will be on the flat side and not the countersunk side.

I find it convenient to drill a hole in a workbench top or a large block of wood so that one end of the hub axle can be inserted in it to hold the hub upright.

Begin by inserting spokes through the upward hub flange. Pass every other one through in the opposite direction. If the hub has countersunk holes, the direction the spokes pass through the holes will be determined by this. The spokes are inserted on the flat, non-countersunk side. If there are no countersunk holes, the choice is up to you. Just make sure that every other spoke passes through in the opposite direction. An easy way to accomplish this is to insert every other spoke, passing them through in the same direction. Then insert the remaining spokes on the same flange, passing them all through in the opposite direction to the first set.

For rear hubs, it's usually necessary to remove the sprocket or sprockets from the hub before the spokes can be passed through the holes in the flange on that side. With clusters of sprockets on freewheels, it's generally easiest to remove the freewheel along with the sprockets rather than the sprockets alone.

When all the spokes on one hub flange are in place, bundle and hold the spokes so they don't fall out and turn the hub over. Position the spokes through the holes in the other flange, using the same placement procedure as for the first flange.

With the hub positioned with one end in the hole in the workbench, position the rim for lacing. Start on the upper hub flange with any spoke that has the end of the spoke facing upward. Group all other spokes in a bundle to the opposite side of the rim. Then turn the rim so that it is positioned with the valve stem hole next to the single spoke you have selected for starting. Insert a spoke nipple into the upper spoke hole that is adjacent to the valve hole.

Depending on the particular rim, this might be either to the right or left of the valve hole. Thread the nipple onto the spoke four full turns. Do the same four thread turns for all spokes. For the time being, assume that the rim will be centered with the hub. Methods for dishing a wheel are detailed later in this section.

Next, select the head-up spoke on either side of the first spoke installed. This will be the second one away, because the next one on each side are head-down spokes. This spoke will go in the fourth (skip three) rim hole from where the first spoke was installed. Continue this pattern until all of the up position spokes on the top hub flange are in position and each is threaded four turns on the nipple. If, for example, the wheel has a total of 36 spokes, nine should now be in place. There should be three vacant rim holes between each spoke that has been installed.

The next step is to twist the hub in the direction that will leave no spoke crossing over the valve stem hole until the spokes are tight. When done correctly, the spoke adjacent to the valve stem hole will angle away from it. Check this carefully, as a mistake here will lead to a spoke being in the way of the valve.

Next, take any spoke in the top flange with the head downward. Move it in the opposite direction of the spokes already in place and cross it over the number of spokes corresponding to the crosses in the spoking pattern being used, generally either three or four. Skip one additional hole in the rim and thread the spoke into the nipple in this rim hole. When done correctly, this will be a top rim hole.

This is the regular spoking pattern. If an interlaced pattern is to be used, the spoke is passed under, rather than over, the last spoke of the crosses.

Regardless of the pattern used, continue with the same plan until all of the spokes with downward facing heads in the top hub flange have been installed with each nipple threaded four turns onto the spoke. When done correctly, the rim will be half laced at this point with a spoke in every other rim hole. The pattern should be consistent. Check this carefully and correct any errors before continuing.

Turn the wheel over. All unlaced spokes should now be on the top hub flange. Take any head-upward spoke on the top hub flange. Then locate the spoke that is head-upward just to the left of this spoke on the bottom flange. Run the top spoke parallel to the bottom one and place it in the hole to the left of that of the bottom spoke. Thread the nipple four turns onto the spoke. When done correctly, the upper and lower spokes with heads upward will follow a consistent pattern, and the distance from the hub to the rim hole will be the same for each spoke because of the offset of the holes on opposite flanges on the hub.

Using this pattern, lace all of the head-upward spokes in the top flange to the rim. If this is done correctly, the pattern around the rim will be consistent with every fourth rim hole empty.

Next, take the remaining spokes in the top flange, which should all have heads downward, and lace them to the rim with the same cross pattern as was used from the other hub flange. If an interlaced pattern is used, don't forget to go under the last spoke in the crosses. The spokes should fit the only vacant rim holes that are in the right positions for the length of the spokes.

If everything is done correctly, the spokes will be in a consistent pattern, will be threaded four turns onto the nipples, and will be of approximately equal tightness. If not, possible causes are a mistake in the spoking pattern, using the wrong cross pattern, or using spokes of the wrong length.

For a rear hub with dishing, the initial lacing is the same, except that different length spokes are used for each hub flange with the shortest length on the sprocket side. A less desirable but still satisfactory method is to use one length of spokes and take care of the dishing by spoke adjustments. Lace the wheel first with four turns on each nipple, as detailed above for a rim that is centered with the hub.

For all wheels, the next step is to tighten all nipples. For a front or centered rear hub and for dished rear hubs where two different lengths of spokes are used, tighten all nipples until the threads on the spokes are just covered. Then tighten all spokes on the other side until about four threads are still visible. The dishing effect is achieved by having the spokes on the sprocket side tighter, and thus shorter than those on the other side. In this way, the wheel will be centered when mounted in the bicycle frame.

Caliper Brakes

The two basic types of caliper brakes are center-pull and side-pull. The center-pull brakes (see Fig. 8-26) consist of a hand lever, cable housing, cable hanger, cable, cable carrier, transverse wire, brake caliper and brake shoes. The side-pull brakes (see Fig. 8-27) consist of a hand lever, cable housing, cable, brake caliper, and brake shoes.

Some hand levers have quick release devices that allow you to open the levers wider than normal, which in turn opens the brake-pad calipers further than usual for easier wheel removals.

To remove a hand lever (Figs. 8-42 and 8-43), first clamp the brake shoes tight against the rim. You can improvise a clamp or use a special tool called a "third hand," which has holes that fit over the nuts on the brake pads and clamp them tightly against the rim.

Some caliper brakes have a quick release for slackening the brake cable. Some center-pull models have a means of disconnecting one end of the transverse cable. If not, loosen the cable at the anchor bolt and pull out enough cable so that the hand lever moves freely. Do not pull the cable completely out of the anchor bolt, as it can be difficult to thread back in. If you are going to remove the cable from the housing anyway, this won't make any difference.

Next, loosen the hand lever clamp. A screwdriver can be used for this. Remove the hand lever from the handlebars.

To make a cable replacement, loosen the anchor bolt on the brake caliper and disconnect the cable. The cable is then pulled out from the hand lever end. On slotted levers, the cable is disconnected from the lever before removal.

The replacement cable should be at least as long as the old one and have the same shaped lead end. When purchasing a new cable, take the old one along to the bicycle shop to make certain you get the right replacement.

Check the cable housing and, if necessary, replace it. Lightly grease the cable. Then thread it through the housing. Connect the cable to the hand lever. Thread the other end of the cable through the anchor bolt. Do not cut off excess cable until after the brakes have been fully adjusted.

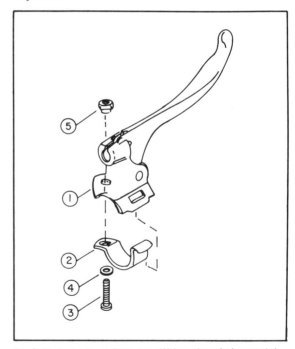

Fig. 8-42. Brake lever. Parts are: (1) lever bracket complete, (2) clamp, (3) lever fixing bolt, (4) lever fixing washer, and (5) lever fixing nut.

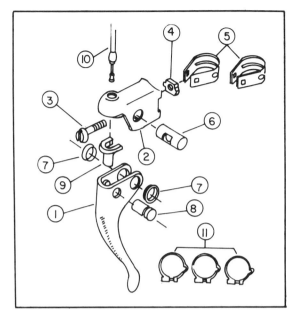

Fig. 8-43. Brake lever. Parts are: (1) lever, (2) lever bracket, (3) pull-up bolt, (4) pull-up nut, (5) clamp, (6) pull-up stud, (7) flanged thrust washer, (8) cable anchor stud, (9) lever adapter, (10) cable set, and (11) outer band for handlebar tubing.

Before adjusting the brakes, first check the brake pads. These wear out from use or harden from age. As a rule, all four brake pads should be replaced at the same time.

You can purchase either the rubber pads separately or the entire brake shoes. The latter are slightly more expensive, but generally worth the difference if the old brake shoes, especially the threads, are even slightly damaged.

Two methods of brake shoe attachment are in common use: a threaded stud on the brake shoe secured to the brake arm by a lock washer and nut, usually an acorn nut; and an un-threaded stud on the brake shoe that fits into an eye bolt on the caliper arm. The latter method, generally used only on center-pull designs, firmly holds the brake shoe in place and permits greater shoe adjustments than the first method.

To make replacements, remove the old brake shoes. If replacing pads only, slide out the old pads and replace them.

Next, install brake shoes on the brake arms. The closed end of the metal holders, if on one end only, should face forward on the bicycle so that the friction against the rim when braking will not force the pads out of the holders.

The first step in making adjustments is to check the alignment of the brake shoes. These should be in line with the edge of the rim. If not, loosen the brake shoe mounting, align the shoe with the rim, and then retighten the mounting. If no adjustment is required, you should still make certain that the brake shoe mountings are tight.

Both brake pads on a caliper should be the same distance from the rim. If not, loosen the caliper mounting nut and turn the calipers until the shoes are both the same distance from the rim. Retighten the caliper mounting nut.

When properly adjusted, the brake pads should be about ⅛-inch from the rims with the hand lever released. In many cases, some adjustment is possible by turning the adjusting barrel. Try this first. If the required adjustment cannot be made in this manner, loosen the anchor cable bolt or cable lock lever. Hold shoes ⅛-inch from the rim, take slack out of the cable by pulling it past the anchor bolt or lever clamp, and then tighten the anchor bolt or lock lever.

Center-pull calipers can ordinarily be cleaned and lubricated without removing the calipers from the bicycle. A second method is to remove the calipers from the bicycle, and clean and lubricate them without disassembling them. Another method is to disassemble, clean, assemble, and lubricate them.

It is often difficult to find replacement parts for inexpensive calipers, and you may have to replace the entire units. Replacement parts are often available for popular brands of more expensive center-pull calipers.

To remove the caliper from a bicycle, loosen the cable anchor bolt and slide the cable free. Unfasten both ends of the transverse cable. Remove the mounting nut and washers and slide the caliper free. If the caliper is to be replaced, try to get the same brand and model.

If you do need to disassemble the caliper, begin by removing the brake shoes. If you do not have assembly drawings for the calipers, make a sketch so that you can get the caliper back together again. Pry loose the spring ends on the brake arms stops. Remove the pivot bolts and separate the brake arms. Remove the springs, marking the left and right side springs, which are not interchangeable.

Clean all parts, except the brake pads, in solvent. Inspect the parts for wear and damage and make replacements as required. Then reassemble in the reverse order. Lightly oil the pivot bolts and holes before installing fasteners. Avoid getting oil on the brake pads. Be careful when installing springs, as they can injure fingers if they slip. Finish by adjusting the brakes, as detailed above.

There are many brands of side-pull calipers in use. Before disassembling calipers to replace worn, broken, or damaged parts, first make certain that replacements are available. If not, you may have to replace the entire unit.

To remove a caliper from a bicycle, loosen the cable anchor bolt and slide the cable free. Remove the mounting nut and washers and slide the caliper free. If you replace a caliper, it often works best to use an exact brand and model replacement.

If you need to disassemble a caliper, begin by removing the brake shoes. If you do not have assembly drawings, make a sketch so that you can assemble the caliper again. Remove the spring ends from the stops on the brake arms, then remove the pivot fasteners. Separate the brake caliper arms.

Clean all parts, except the brake pads, in solvent. Inspect for wear and damage and make replacements as required. Reassemble in reverse order. Lightly oil the pivot bolts and holes before installing the fasteners. Finish by adjusting the brakes as detailed above in this section.

Common caliper brake problems include:

- Sticking brakes caused by a bent caliper part or hand lever, or a cable sticking in the housing because of damaged housing. The problem can often be corrected by bending parts slightly and/or applying lubrication.
- Dragging brake pad. First, check the shoe adjustments. The caliper should be centered when released. Dragging brake pads can also be caused by a loose mounting nut or sticking pivots. In some cases, the problem is caused by the wheel being out of alignment.

- Cable frequently breaks. Usually, some part of the cable housing is chafing. Check for burrs, bends, and kinks in the cable housing. Replace the housing.

Pedals

Pedals that cannot be taken apart are generally the least expensive. They can be lubricated externally by squirting oil on the bearings. If they break down, they are usually discarded and replaced with new ones, often of a type that can be disassembled.

To remove pedals that cannot be disassembled, it is important to note that left side pedals have left hand spindle threads. Turn clockwise to remove them. These are generally marked "L" on the threaded end of the spindle. Right side pedals have conventional right hand spindle threads and are marked "R". Turn them counterclockwise to remove them.

If you want to overhaul rubber pad pedals that can be disassembled, first remove the pedals from the bicycle. To disassemble a pedal, remove the nuts from the long bolts that extend through the rubber pedal pads and slip the pedal pads, bolts, and dust cap off as a unit. You only need to take this apart if replacement of any parts is necessary, such as the rubber pads.

Next, clamp the pedal spindle in a vise. Remove the lock nut, key washer, and bearing cone. The two types of bearings commonly used are loose ball bearings and bearings mounted in retainers. Remove the bearings, bearing cup, spindle housing, inner bearing cup, and inner bearings.

Clean all parts, except the rubber pedal pads, in solvent. Replace parts as required. If there is major damage to an inexpensive pedal, it may be less expensive to purchase a new pedal than replacement parts.

When reassembling the pedal, add bicycle grease to the bearings. Hand tighten the bearing cone against the bearings. Then back off a quarter turn. Keep the cone in this position, slip on the key washer, and then thread on the lock nut and tighten it.

To disassemble rattrap pedals, remove the pedal from the bicycle. Remove the pedal spindle cap. This might be threaded on or held in place with small bolts. Remove the locknut.

Slip off the keyed lockwasher. Thread off the cone and collect the loose bearings or remove the caged bearing assembly. Slide off the pedal body. Collect the loose inner bearings or remove the caged bearing assembly. Clean all parts in solvent. Inspect for wear and damage and replace parts as required. When assembling, hold loose bearings in pedal body cup with grease. The pedal body should be positioned with the inner cup upright. Slip the spindle in place. Hold it firmly against the bearings and turn the pedal over. Install bearings in grease in the outer cup. Install the cone. Assembly is, of course, greatly simplified on pedals with the bearings in retainers.

Finger tighten the cone, then back off about a quarter turn. Install the keyed lock washer and locknut. Install the pedal spindle cap after checking to make certain that the pedal turns freely without end play. If not, make necessary cone adjustments.

While most rattrap pedals are lubricated with grease, some expensive racing pedals use oil. These require more frequent servicing, but have the advantage of less friction.

Toe Clips, Straps, and Cleats

Toe clips and straps are commonly used only on rattrap pedals with saw-tooth notches to prevent shoes from slipping. Racing pedals often do not have the saw-tooth notches, and special cleated shoes are used.

Pedals with toe clips and straps can be purchased with the clips and straps already attached to the pedals, or you can purchase clips and straps that will fit most rattrap pedals. Toe clips are bolted to the pedals, and straps pass through notches in most rattrap pedals.

Straps are available with buckles and quick release attachments. Toe clips are sometimes used alone, but most often the clips and straps are used together.

From time to time, the straps might require replacement. The clips generally have a long life span.

Chains

The chains used on single-speed and multi-speed hub geared bicycles are usually classified as "wide" and those on derailleur and single-speed track bicycles as "narrow." Wide chain is ⅛-inch wide, the width of the rollers, and usually has a ½-inch *pitch*, the distance between the centers of the rivets. Wide chains employ a master link for joining the ends together.

Narrow chains also have a ½-inch pitch, but have only a 3/32-inch (2.38 mm) width. These are connected at all links by rivets. Master links are not used on chains for derailleur gears, as the extra width will not pass through the derailleur mechanisms or fit between the sprockets of the cluster.

To remove a wide chain, loosen the rear hub axle nuts and slide the hub forward to slacken the chain. Locate the master link, which is wider than a normal link. Flex the chain and pry the master link off with a screwdriver. Remove the link posts and backing plate. These slide out as a unit.

A rivet extractor tool is required to remove a narrow chain, either the screw type and the plier type. Regardless of the type used, open the extractor tool and slip it over the chain. Line it up with a rivet and then close the extractor until the rivet is free of all but the last plate. Do not drive the rivet all the way out.

Remove the extractor tool. The chain can then be separated. After removal, clean the chain by soaking it in solvent. A stiff brush can also be used. Allow the chain to dry.

To lubricate the chain, soak it in a pan of bicycle chain oil. Then hang the chain up, preferably overnight, and allow it to drip dry over a collecting pan. After the chain has dripped dry, use a cloth to remove any remaining excess oil. The chain is then ready to be reinstalled on the bicycle.

To install a wide chain, place the chain over the front and rear sprocket teeth. Insert the backing plate with two posts in chain holes to join the ends of the chain. Position the master link and bend the chain toward you. Snap the link in place. Reposition the rear hub and tighten the axle nuts. The chain should have approximately ½-inch slack in it when properly adjusted. If not, loosen the axle nuts and readjust. Make certain that the wheel is centered between the frame drop-outs.

To install a narrow chain, the extended rivet should face away from the bicycle. Feed this end of the chain around the smallest chainwheel at the crank. Feed the other end around the smallest rear sprocket and through jockey and idler pulleys. Bring the two ends together and use the chain tool for driving the rivet back into position.

A broken or defective link in both narrow and wide chain can be replaced by driving out the rivets with a chain tool. Replace the links and, if necessary, the rivets. Use the same tool to drive the rivets back in. Rivets can be started into a side plate by holding them in position with needle-nosed pliers and tapping them in place.

On a wide chain, a defective link can also be replaced with a master link. Use an extractor tool to remove a defective link.

Adjustments in chain length can be made in a similar manner. When selecting a new chain, use the same length as the old chain.

Tight links are frequently a problem when a chain is not oiled periodically. If bicycle chain oil will not cure the problem, use a rivet extractor tool to move the rivets of sticking links slightly to one side and then back into position again. A freeing oil can also be used to advantage here. Apply the oil and then use tool to move the rivet to one side and then back again.

If side plates are bent or if the above steps will not cure the sticking, install new links to replace the sticking ones. If many links stick, it's usually best to get a new chain.

Crank Sets

A crank set consists of an axle, crank or pedal arms, a chain wheel and the necessary bearings, cups, washers, and locking devices to hold everything in place in the bottom bracket of the bicycle frame.

Three basic types of crank-axle assemblies are used on modern bicycles: one-piece steel forged axle and cranks in a single unit, as shown in Fig. 8-28; cottered crank assemblies, which have pedal or crank arms attached to a separate axle by means of cotters (Fig. 8-29); and cotterless crank assemblies with the crank arms drawn onto wedged ends of the axle with crank bolts (Fig. 8-44).

The axles for both the cottered and cotterless assemblies are almost always steel. The pedal arms for the cottered assemblies are generally steel. The pedal arms for the cotterless assemblies are usually lightweight aluminum alloy.

The basic procedure for overhauling crank sets is to disassemble, clean, inspect, replace parts as required, lubricate, and then reassemble.

One-piece crank sets can be disassembled by removing the chain guard and chain. Remove both pedals. The threads on the left pedal are left-hand threads, so turn the pedal spindle clockwise to remove it. The pedal on the chainwheel side is turned counterclockwise for removal.

Remove the lock nut on the left side of the crank. This has a left-hand thread, so it is turned clockwise for loosening. The required leverage can be gained by using a wrench on the lock nut while holding the crank arm with one hand. After the lock nut is clear of the threads, slide it off over the pedal arm.

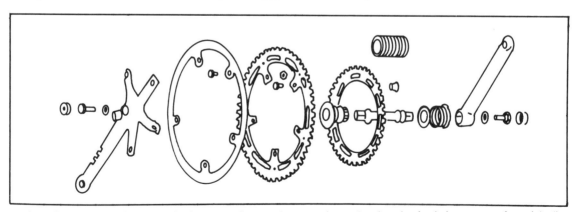

Fig. 8-44. Cotterless crank assemblies have crank arms drawn on to wedged ends of axle by means of crank bolts.

Remove the keyed lock washer. Then remove the adjusting cone by turning it counterclockwise with a screwdriver in one of the slots. When the adjusting cone is clear of the threads, slide it off over the pedal arm.

Slide out the bearing and retainer assembly. Unless worn or damaged, the hanger cups need not be removed. If you need to remove them, use a wood dowel and drive them out from the opposite side. The crank can now be slipped out on the sprocket side of the frame. Remove the bearing and retainer assembly from the sprocket side.

If it's necessary to remove the chainwheel from the crank, remove the stationary cone. The sprocket can then be removed. ·

Clean parts in solvent. Inspect all parts for wear and damage. Replace parts as required. Reassembly is basically the reverse of disassembly, except that bicycle grease is added to the bearings and cups. The adjusting cone is tightened until the cranks still turn freely, but without play. Then install the keyed lock washer and lock nut, firmly tightening the lock nut. Install chain, chain guard, and pedals.

With the bicycle in a maintenance rack or with the back of the bicycle held off the floor, work the cranks. They should turn freely and have almost no play. If not, remove the lock nut and lock washer and readjust the cone.

For cottered crank assemblies, disassembly begins by removing the cotters with a special cotter tool. First, remove the nut and lock washer from the cotter. Open the jaws of the cotter removal tool. Position the tool and turn the handle to drive the cotter out. The same tool can also be used to set cotters.

If the special tool is not available, the cotters can be driven out with a hammer. This method leaves much to be desired, however, and damage to cotters frequently results.

To use the hammer method, loosen the nut on the cotter until it is flush with the end of the cotter. Place the pedal arm on a bench or block so that tapping out the cotter will not place stress on the bearings or axle. A block of wood can be used between the hammer and the cotter, but a single, sharp tap directly to the cotter with the hammer head often works just as well.

After the cotter has been removed, work the crank arm free of the axle. On the chainwheel side, the chainwheel will come off with the crank arm. Some chainwheels are permanently fixed to the pedal crank; others can be disassembled by removing mounting bolts.

After both crank arms have been removed, unfasten the lock ring from the left side with a special hook spanner tool. If you don't have one, you can get by with a punch and hammer, although this is poor technique and leaves much to be desired.

Next, remove the adjusting cup with a wrench by turning it counterclockwise. Some models require a peg spanner wrench. Some crank sets have loose bearings and others have bearings in a retainer. If you are uncertain about yours, be prepared to catch loose bearings. Take the adjusting cup all the way off. If the bearings are in a retainer, remove it from the assembly. The axle can now be pulled out from the left side of the bottom bracket. Next, remove the stationary cup on the right-hand side. If bearings are not in a retainer, catch them. If the bearings are in a retainer, remove this from the housing.

Clean all parts in solvent. Inspect parts for wear and damage, and replace parts as necessary.

For reassembly, reverse the order of steps for disassembly, except that lubrication is applied to the bearings. Loose bearings can be held in place in grease during the assembly. Tweezers are handy for placing the bearings. The adjusting cup should be tightened until the axle turns freely with only a trace of end play. Install and tighten the lock ring.

The best way to seat cotters is with a cotter tool. Position the crank arm on the axle and the cotter in the hole. Position the cotter tool and then tighten until the cotter is firmly set. If you do not have a cotter tool, a substitute method is to position a block of wood so that stress will not be placed on bearings or axle. Tap the cotter with a hammer to seat it. Install the lock washer and nut and tighten down.

Make certain that cotters are firmly seated because, this is a frequent source of trouble. A slight play between the axle and pedal arm will quickly lead to wear and damage. It's a good idea to check this again after the bicycle has been ridden.

Overhaul is basically the same for the

cotterless assembly as for the cottered, except for the method of attachment and removal of the pedal arms from the axle. The procedure for the removal of crank arms is the same for both arms. Begin by removing the dust cap. Some models require an Allen wrench and others a wide-blade screwdriver. Next, remove the crank or spindle bolts. A socket wrench or special wrench designed especially for this purpose. Hold the crank arm in one hand and work the wrench on the bolt with the other hand.

A special cotterless crank extractor tool is used to remove the crank from the axle. Some of these have their own handles; others are turned with a wrench. Regardless, the extractor is screwed into the dust cap threads. Turning the tool then applies pressure against the end of the axle and forces the crank arm off. For the remainder of the disassembly, follow the steps outlined above for cottered crank assemblies. After cleaning the parts, inspect for damage and wear and replace parts as required. Lubrication and axle assembly in the bottom bracket is the same as for cottered crank sets.

The crank arms can be positioned in any of four directions, but make sure the two arms face opposite directions. The crank or spindle bolts should be tightened securely and then checked after a short ride. For the first 150 miles of riding, retighten the bolts every 50 miles. If a bicycle is ridden with loose crank bolts or with crank arms that are not firmly seated, damage will usually result.

For all types of crank assemblies, inspect the parts for wear and damage after cleaning the parts in solvent, as follows:

- Inspect the axle to make certain it is not bent. This is rarely a problem on one-piece cranks.
- Pedal arm straightness is best check before disassembly with the pedals still in place. Any untrueness will show up while riding because the pedal centers will not be parallel to the axle.
- Check all threads. Parts with stripped or damaged threads, unless extremely minor, should be replaced.
- Bearings and cones should be smooth and unpitted. It is generally best to replace all bearings at the same time regardless of

whether the bearings are loose or in a retainer.
- Check chainwheels for bent teeth. These can sometimes be straightened, but usually the chainwheels will have to be replaced.
- Check all other parts. Especially important are cotters, axle notches for cotters, and cotter holes through the crank arms. Early replacement of parts can often prevent more costly repairs later.

Derailleurs

The basic principles of derailleur gear systems were covered above. For adjusting and overhauling derailleurs, place the bicycle in a maintenance rack or turn the bicycle upside down. Make certain that brake cables or other parts of the bicycle will not be damaged. You can construct a wooden frame with notches for the handlebars to hold the bicycle upright and protect the brake cables. While it is generally most convenient to have the bicycle right side up, the most important thing is to be able to turn the pedal cranks by hand and work the gear shift controls.

Adjusting Rear Derailleurs. A common problem is slack in the control cable. The cables tend to stretch with use, and the cable no longer pulls the derailleur cage all the way to the largest sprocket. In turn, a cable that is too tight won't allow the cable to release far enough for the derailleur mechanism spring to pull the cage back to the smallest sprocket.

Minor adjustments to the cable can be made by unscrewing the cable where it joins the derailleur mechanism if it is too slack or tightening it if the cable is too tight. If this will not go far enough to make the required correction, or the particular derailleur has no adjustment barrel, loosen the cable clamp nut and loosen or tighten the cable as required. Then retighten the cable clamp nut.

If there is enough slack in the cable when the control lever is released (pushed as far forward as it will go), and the derailleur still will not return to the cage so the chain will derail to the smallest sprocket, the problem might be sticking pivots in the derailleur mechanism.

Adjust by oiling the pivot points on the derailleur mechanism.

The control cable must slide through the housing freely to allow the derailleur spring to pull the derailleur cage to the smallest sprocket. If the cable does not move freely in the housing, try adding a few drops of light bicycle oil to each end of the cable at the entrances to the housing. If this does not cure the problem, remove the cable from the housing. First, disconnect the cable from the derailleur. Then disconnect the cable from the control lever and pull it out of the housing. If the cable is rusty or appears damaged, replace it with a new one. Otherwise, apply a light coating of bicycle grease to the original wire and reinstall it in the housing. If the cable still will not slide freely, the problem might be in the housing. Replace the housing if necessary.

When selecting housings or cables, take the old ones along with you to the bicycle shop so that you can get exact replacements. New cables should be at least as long as the original and have the same type of end fitting for connection to the control lever.

Apply a light coating of bicycle grease before inserting the cable into the housing. Turn the cable while threading it into the housing. Connect the cable to the control lever. Pass the other end of the cable through the anchor bolt. Adjust the cable length and tighten. Do not cut off any excess cable until all adjustments have been made and everything is working properly. Always leave enough extra cable for future adjustments. It's a good idea to cap the end of the cable so that it will not unravel. Caps are available at bicycle shops.

The same procedure is used for replacing cables and housing for front derailleurs.

Returning to the rear derailleur, with the control cable working smoothly and adjusted to the correct length and the derailleur mechanism pivot points oiled, the next step is to consider the range adjustments on the rear derailleur.

Range Adjustment. This is accomplished by stop adjusting screws that limit the travel inward and outward of the derailleur cage. If the low gear screw (marked with an "L" on most derailleurs) is too far out, the chain can go past the largest sprocket. If there is no spoke guard, it can damage the spokes. If the low gear adjustment screw is too far in, the derailleur cage cannot guide the chain to the largest sprocket.

If the high gear screw (marked on most derailleurs with an "H") is too far out, the chain can pass the lowest gear and go between the smallest sprocket and the bicycle frame. When the screw is too far in, the chain cannot reach the smallest sprocket.

When you make adjustments, the control lever should be in the extreme forward (slack cable) position for making high gear adjustments and in the back (tension) position for making low gear adjustments.

If the derailleur tends to jump out of set gear, the problem is most likely in the pressure plate adjustment of the control lever. Check to make sure that oil has not gotten on the pressure plate. If oil is present, disassemble and clean the pressure plate in solvent. Dry and reassemble. Adjustment of the pressure plate is made by tightening the screw to increase friction and loosening to decrease it. Wing screws are used on many control levers for easy adjustments.

If shifting is difficult even though the control cable is properly adjusted and working freely, the chain cage might be bent out of line. If so, you may be able to straighten it by bending it back in line. Take care not to bend the mounting plate on the bicycle frame, however. This generally isn't a problem on derailleurs that attach on the axle bolts.

Adjusting Front Derailleurs. To make adjustments to front derailleurs (in addition to making adjustments with the limit screws), the derailleur unit can be repositioned up or down and twisted at its mounts.

First, check the cable and housing. Follow the same procedures as given above for rear derailleur controls. When the cable is working properly, adjust its length. Then make adjustments as required with the two adjustment screws for limit of cage travel. On most front derailleurs, cable tension moves the cage outward to the largest chainwheel. Spring action in the derailleur mechanism pulls the cage inward when the tension is released. A few front derailleurs work the opposite of this.

Oil all pivots so that they move freely. This is a frequent source of difficulty.

It might be necessary to reposition the front derailleur mechanism on its mounts. The following conditions must be met:

—The chain guide is parallel to the chainwheels.

—When the chain is on the largest front chainwheel and largest rear sprocket, it does not touch the chain guide.

—When the chain is on the smallest front chainwheel and smallest rear sprocket, it does not touch the chain guide.

—The chain guide clears the largest front chainwheel by about ⅛-inch.

The chain is frequently responsible for derailleur shifting problems. A tight chain link can cause difficulties. (Methods of freeing tight chain links are covered above.)

Problems can also occur from worn chain and bent or worn sprocket teeth. This might require replacement of the chain or sprockets.

The rear axle might be angled in the frame and cause rear sprockets to be out of alignment. Loosen the rear axle nuts or quick release devices, straighten the wheel in the frame, and retighten the axle mounts.

For routine overhaul of rear derailleurs, the unit itself need not be disassembled. To remove a rear derailleur from the bicycle, first remove the chain. Disconnect the shift cable from the rear derailleur. Loosen the mounting bolt or nut and remove the derailleur unit from the bicycle frame.

Clean the derailleur unit in solvent. Inspect the unit for wear and damage. Inexpensive derailleurs are often replaced as a unit when worn or damaged. On more expensive units, the mechanism can be disassembled and defective parts replaced, provided that the needed parts are available.

Lubricate pivot points and pulley wheels with bicycle oil. Reinstall the unit on the bicycle and adjust as detailed above.

For routine overhauls of front derailleurs, it isn't necessary to disassemble the front derailleur unit. To remove the front derailleur from the bicycle, remove the chain and disconnect the shift cable from the front derailleur unit. Unfasten the mounting bolts. Remove the derailleur unit from the bicycle frame. Clean the derailleur in solvent. Inspect for damage and

wear. Ordinarily, the unit need not be disassembled unless part replacements are necessary. Oil the pivot points and reinstall the unit on the bicycle. Adjust as described above.

Derailleur control levers are located on down tubes (Fig. 8-45) handlebar stems (Fig. 8-46), handlebar ends (Fig. 8-47), and elsewhere. Shifter disassembly is generally simple. Remove the lever fixing bolt, and the parts slide off. If you don't have the assembly drawings make drawings as you take parts off so that you can reassemble them. Clean all parts in solvent and wipe with a clean cloth. Replace bent, broken, and worn parts as required. Do not apply lubrication, because friction is necessary to prevent the lever from slipping. After overhaul and adjustments, make a final check with the bicycle in a maintenance rack. Run through the gear changes a number of times. Gear changes should work smoothly.

Head Sets and Handlebars

The head set (see Fig. 8-22) allows the steering mechanism to pivot. It consists of the bearings, cups, cones, and necessary fastening and locking devices for holding the fork head or stem in the frame head tube. When assembled, the only direct connection between the fork and the frame are the bearings. This allows the fork to turn in the head tube. The handlebar post mounts inside the fork head or stem. The handlebar post usually extends upward and then angles forward to the clamp that holds the handlebars.

To overhaul a head set, the first step is to remove the handlebar post from the fork stem. Two types of handlebar post wedges in common use are external wedge and internal wedge. The external type places all the stress on one side of the fork head. It is less desirable than the internal type, which better distributes the stress on the inside of the fork head.

Both types are disassembled from the fork head in the same way. First, loosen the stem bolt a few turns. Avoid continuing to turn it until it comes out of the wedge. Next, with a block of wood over the bolt head, tap the block with a hammer. Remove the handlebar post from the fork head by twisting slightly back and forth while pulling upward on it. Use liquid wrench to help free it if it is rusted in place.

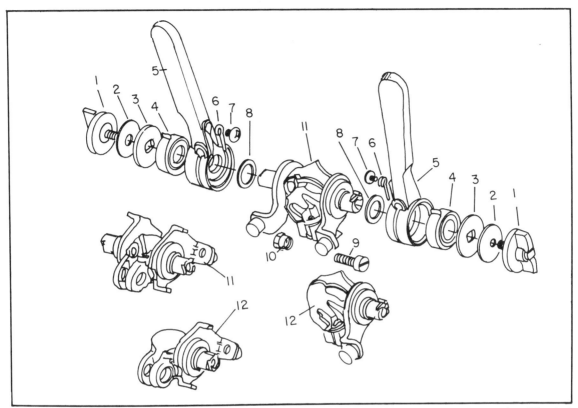

Fig. 8-45. Shifting levers for down tube. Parts are: (1) wing bolt, (2) coned disk spring, (3) non-turn washer, (4) spiral spring, (5) lever, (6) leaf spring, (7) screw, (8) washer, (9) clamp bolt, (10) clamp nut, (11) level clamp for 10-speed, and (12) lever clamp for 5-speed.

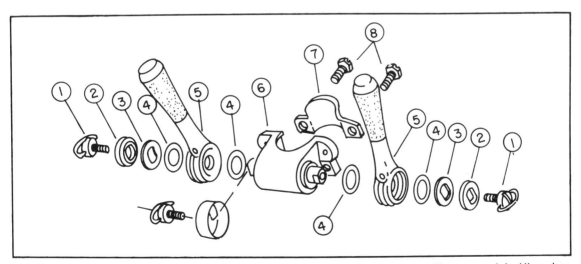

Fig. 8-46. Shifting levers for handlebar stem. Parts are: (1) wing screw, (2) non-turn washer, (3) pressure plate, (4) washer, (5) lever, (6) lever frame, (7) clamp plate, and (8) clamp bolt.

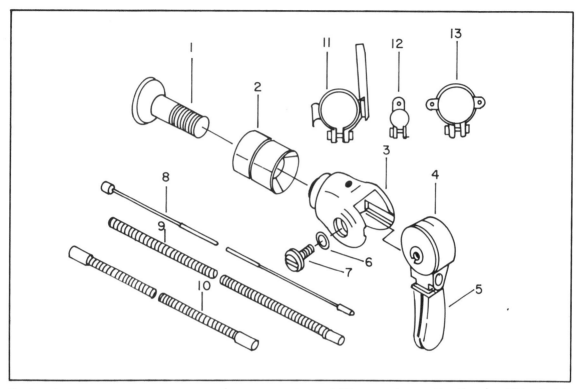

Fig. 8-47. Shifting lever for handlebar ends. Parts are: (1) anchor bolt, (2) segment assembly with spring, (3) body, (4) lever assembly with lever cap, (5) lever cap, (6) spring washer, (7) lever fixing bolt, (8) inner cable, (9) lever end outer casing, (10) outer casing, (11) cable guide, (12) outer stopper, and (13) outer stopper.

Remove the lock nut from the head set with a wrench. On caliper brake bicycles, slip off the brake cable collar guide. Remove the lock ring or washer. Use a wrench to remove the adjusting cup, turning it counterclockwise until it is free of the fork head.

If the bearings are loose, remove them from the upper stationary cone. Then, holding the fork in the frame, turn the frame over. Pull the fork from the frame. The crown cone will normally stay on the fork. Remove the loose bearings. If the bearings are in retainers, pull the fork out of the frame and remove the retainers and bearings from the stationary cones.

You will not need to remove stationary cones from the frame head tube unless they require replacement. If you need to remove them, use a wooden dowel and carefully drive them out from the inside of the frame head tube. The crown cone can be removed by sliding it off the fork head.

Next, clean all parts in solvent. Inspect for wear and damage and make replacements as required.

Reassembly is essentially the reverse of disassembly, except that bicycle grease is added to the bearings. In the case of loose bearings, begin assembly by turning the bicycle frame upside down. Apply grease to the lower stationary cone. Insert the fork head part way in the frame head tube. Place individual bearings in grease. Tweezers are good for handling the bearings. Slip the fork the rest of the way into the head tube and hold it firmly in position while turning the frame upright. Fill the upper stationary cone with grease and position the individual bearings. The adjusting cup should be tightened until the fork still rotates freely, but without end play. When this has been achieved, install remaining parts of the head set. Adjust the handlebar post to desired height, but make certain that at least 2½ inches remain inside the fork head, which is necessary for safety.

Straight and upright handlebars commonly have rubber or plastic hand grips. These sometimes require replacement. If you cannot twist the old handlebar grips off by hand, cut them off with a sharp knife. Glue the new handlebar grips on with rim or gasket cement, and use a cloth to clean off excess cement.

Dropped handlebars are commonly taped. The tape can be cloth, plastic, or rubber. Begin wrapping about 3 inches from the clamp in the center of the handlebars. Work outward, pulling the tape tight and overlapping about a ¼-inch. Either skip over or take a wrap around the caliper brake handle mountings. At the end of the handlebar, run the tape off the end and cut it off, leaving a couple of inches of extra tape on the end. Stuff the end of the tape inside the end of the handlebar and install either a push-in plug or an expansion bolted plug.

Saddles and Saddle Posts

A well designed saddle and saddle post assembly is relatively trouble-free. It is important to select a good saddle to start with and adjust it properly. Most regular saddles can be adjusted within a limited range for height, angle, and forward/backward position. The saddle can also be turned so that it doesn't point straight forward, if that's necessary. In addition, many saddles have a tension adjustment.

Height adjustment is usually made by loosening the seat post clamp at the top of the frame seat tube, adjusting the seat post up or down to the desired height, and then retightening the clamp bolt. There are also wedge-type seat posts that are held in place like handlebar posts. To adjust, loosen the bolt on top of the post about four turns. Tap to drive the wedge loose. Adjust height and retighten the bolt. A major problem with this type of saddle post is that the saddle often has to be removed to get at the adjustment bolt.

For safety, it is generally recommended that at least 2½ inches of the saddle post be down in the seat tube of the frame. If this does not give you the required height, replace the saddle post with a longer one.

The saddle post clamp generally allows you to adjust both forward/backward position and angle of saddle. Loosen the clamp. The saddle can then be slid forward or backwards. The normal adjustment is with the front of the saddle about 2 inches behind the crank center. Normal tilt is within one notch of the level position, but some riders prefer a more exaggerated tilt. Retighten the clamp when the saddle is positioned the way you want it. Some of the more expensive alloy posts have a saddle bracket that can be adjusted more precisely.

Some saddles have tension adjustments that allow you to tighten or slacken the saddle top by turning a nut under the saddle.

Some saddles have plastic or rubber covers or complete tops that can be replaced when they wear out. Other saddles have to be replaced completely, although on more expensive saddles the mounting clamp need not be replaced. Inexpensive saddles generally only come with the clamp included.

RECONDITIONING BICYCLES

In many cases, you can save considerable money by purchasing a used bicycle in run-down condition and restoring it for exercise and physical fitness riding.

The Frame

To build a good bicycle, you need a sound frame. Don't worry about the finish, because painting will take care of this. The important thing is that the frame is straight, undamaged, and of sufficient quality that the finished bicycle will be suitable for your riding purposes. In some cases, a damaged frame can be repaired, but generally this is only practical if the damage is extremely minor or cosmetic. Check especially the frame joints. A minor fracture in a welded or brazed joint can be repaired by taking the frame to a commercial shop if you don't have the skill and/or equipment to do this work yourself. It's generally safest to use brazing rather than welding. The lower heat of brazing usually has less adverse effects on the tensile strength of the steel.

A bent frame can be a more serious matter. Even minor damage can be difficult to correct without special tools. Well-equipped bicycle shops usually have a number of special tools and devices for straightening and aligning frames. Without these, you will be extremely limited. If the frame is high quality and worth the expense, I suggest that you take the frame to a bicycle shop and have it straightened and aligned for you.

If you do want to attempt frame straightening yourself, it usually works best if you do it with props and application of hand, foot, or steady prying pressure rather than by using a hammer. A badly bent fork can be replaced with a new or used one, but the replacement should be the same size and shape as the original. Not all forks will fit all frames.

Regardless of whether or not you intend to paint the frame, I suggest that all components be disassembled, cleaned, overhauled, and replaced. If the frame does not require repainting, this can be done one component at a time. If the frame will be painted, strip all components off, including the fork. It is nearly impossible to do a good painting job with the components in place, even with careful masking.

Painting

Painting is both an art and craft. Most bicycle owners who want to paint their own bicycles are hampered by lack of professional equipment and a dust free painting environment with controlled temperature and humidity and good lighting. With care, however, a reasonably good paint job can be done.

The first step is to disassemble all components from the frame, including bearing cups from the bottom bracket and head tubes. While it is possible to paint with the fork still mounted in the frame, I suggest you remove the fork and paint the frame and fork separately. You will probably want to disassemble the head set for overhaul anyway.

You may also want to paint other parts of the bicycle, such as fenders, chain guards, and rims. It's generally best to have each part separate for painting.

Whether or not you need to remove all of the old paint depends on its condition, the type of paint you intend to apply and, to a certain extent, the colors of the old and new paint. If the old paint peels away when you try to sand it, then it will probably have to be removed. Since putty is often used to fill nicks and dents on manufactured bicycles, I suggest that you re-

move paint by fine sanding rather than with paint remover, because most paint removers tend to remove fillers, too. If you do use a paint remover, be prepared to apply new putty.

Many home paint jobs look amateurish because of inadequate surface preparation. In general, don't expect the paint to fill defects. Avoid using coarse grades of sandpaper; start with medium grades and work up to fine.

You must decide what type of paint you want to use: lacquer, enamel, acrylic, epoxy, or whatever. Use only paint designed for metal surfaces and make certain that it is compatible with old paint if the frame is not stripped bare. Once you have decided on the type of paint, you will need to get filler and primer, if required, that is compatible with the paint selected.

Spray painting will generally provide the smoothest finish, but only if you have the necessary equipment and painting know-how. Also, without adequate safety precautions, spray painting can be extremely hazardous to your health.

The common alternative is to use paint in spray cans, but these have similar or even greater health hazards. My own recommendation is that you avoid these, as it is almost impossible to avoid breathing the fumes, even if you paint outdoors, without expensive respirators.

The alternative is brush painting. If you get the right kind of paint, a good job can be done in this manner.

After the frame and all other components have been sanded and are ready for painting, position them for applying the paint. Good lighting and a dust free area are important, but for safety reasons, I suggest that the painting be done outdoors. Do the painting on a dry, warm (but not hot) day in a shaded area out of direct sunlight.

If primer is required, apply and allow to dry. Additional light sanding may be required before the application of the finish coat or coats of paint. Follow the paint manufacturer's recommendations regarding drying times between costs. Allow the paint to thoroughly dry before reassembling the bicycle.

Cleaning Plate Components

Pits and bubbles of rust can be removed from

plated metal surfaces by light rubbing with a slightly abrasive cleaning pad, followed by metal cleaner, polish, and finally wax. In many cases, parts that look quite bad can be restored to good appearance in this manner. You can also have parts chrome-plated at commercial shops. I suggest that you paint over plated surfaces only as a last resort. If this is done, the plating will usually have to be completely removed to give the paint a good bonding surface.

Assembly

Before assembly, clean, inspect, and replace parts as detailed above. The wheels may require trueing. In many cases, it's advisable to replace bearings throughout and wires in control cables. After assembly is complete, make final adjustments, and the bicycle is ready for use.

Chapter 9

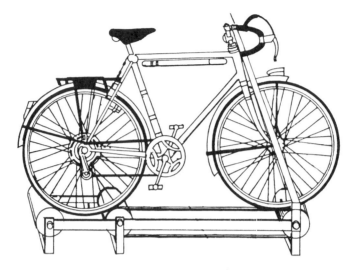

Stationary Bicycles

A VARIETY OF STATIONARY EXERCISE PEDAL CYCLES is available, but only those that make you do the work are of proven value. This type simulates riding an actual bicycle—at least the pedaling part of bicycle riding. You pedal against a resistance, which in many cases can be adjusted for various workloads. In my opinion, exercise pedal cycles that rock you back and forth while you pedal are of little value. Even worse are those with motors. Passive or active resistance to pedals that are turned by a motor is not the same thing as doing the work yourself.

The lowest cost models are built with components similar to those used on children's tricycles and generally lack both the precision and durability to be of much use as exercise machines. Quality models generally cost $100 or more when purchased new, but you can often buy a used model for a fraction of this. An alternative is to build your own from used bicycle components, as detailed below.

STATIONARY CYCLING

Being able to pedal a bicycle in one place without going anywhere has many applications for exercising, training, and physical fitness testing. While a number of stationary exercise pedal cycles are on the market, and you can even construct your own, as detailed later, you will probably want to first consider using a regular bicycle on rollers or a special stand for bicycling in one place.

There are two basic types of bicycle rollers that allow you to use regular bicycles for stationary pedaling: those with a roller for the rear wheel and a frame stand to support the bicycle; and those with three rollers, two for the rear wheel and one for the front wheel, with the bicycle either free or supported.

For general exercise training, I recommend that the bicycle be fully supported. This allows you to exercise without having to worry about falling. Riding free of support on rollers most closely simulates actual bicycle riding and is often used for training for bicycle racing. Because there is danger of falling, however, I do not recommend this method for general exercise and physical fitness work.

A number of stands with a single roller, such as the design shown in Fig. 9-1, are on the

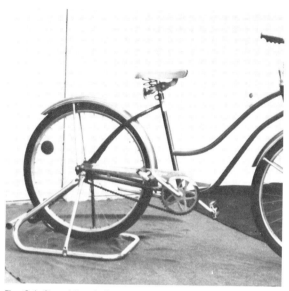

Fig. 9-1. Stand for stationary cycling on regular bicycle.

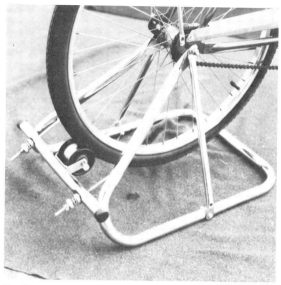

Fig. 9-2. A roller wheel provides resistance.

market. These attach to the bicycle, usually to the rear axle but sometimes elsewhere, and hold the bicycle upright in a position so that the rear wheel turns on a roller (Fig. 9-2). On many designs, it's the rider's weight that provides most of the resistance, although some models have a means of adjusting the resistance to a greater level. Also, tire inflation often changes the resistance, with a larger inflation pressure giving less resistance.

You can also construct your own roller stand, as shown in Fig. 9-3. A boat trailer roller is used. A variation is to use two rollers for the rear wheel of the bicycle, as shown in Fig. 9-4.

Regardless of whether you buy or build, the stand can be attached and removed from the bicycle, allowing you to use the same bicycle for both stationary exercising and on-the-road training. These stands and rollers can be used with single-speed and multi-speed bicycles and

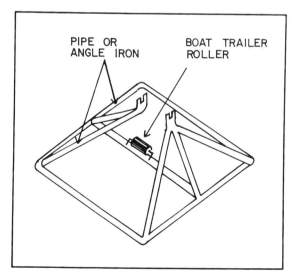

Fig. 9-3. Construction plan for roller stand with one roller.

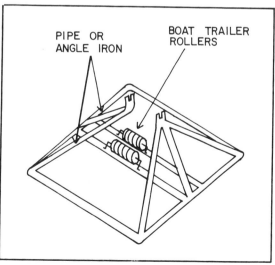

Fig. 9-4. Construction plan for roller stand with two rollers.

allow gear shifting in the same manner as regular cycling.

A three-roller arrangement for stationary bicycling is shown in Fig. 9-5. A drive belt runs from the forward rear-wheel roller to the front roller to turn the front bicycle wheel to more closely simulate actual bicycle riding. A stand for holding the bicycle upright can be added, as shown. This is a somewhat expensive way of obtaining essentially the same effect, except for the turning front wheel, as the simple stands described above.

A variety of manufactured three-roller assemblies are available, or you can construct your own. Regardless, I suggest that you use a support stand to hold the bicycle upright so that you can exercise without the danger of falling.

MANUFACTURED MODELS

When selecting a new exercise cycle, here are some points to consider:

□ The cycle should pedal smoothly and the resistance be adjustable through a wide range of workloads. Pedal cycles with motors are essentially useless: if you want exercise, you need to do the work yourself—actively and not just passively with your legs being pulled around by a motor. Also, I do not recommend the cycles where the saddle and handles rock back and forth as you pedal, as these distract from the continuous pedaling action that is so important for physical fitness exercise.

□ The saddle should feel comfortable and be adjustable to desired height. Many manufactured models feature wide saddles, which can be positioned fairly low. This can be okay, since wind resistance isn't a factor, but there are advantages to having a narrow saddle positioned high enough so that your legs will be nearly extended at the low points in the pedal cycles. On many manufactured stationary exercise pedal cycles, it is a simple matter to switch to a narrow saddle, although in some cases it will be necessary to also change to a longer saddle post to give the necessary height.

□ Features on manufactured models include speedometers mileage indicators, timers, adjustable pedal resistance control dials, and foot straps. These all have useful applications for exercising, as they allow you control and monitor your exercise workloads.

□ Resistance is provided in three main ways: by a resistance wheel that turns against the cycle wheel, (Fig. 9-6), by

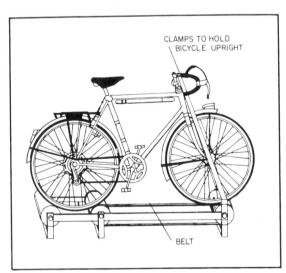

Fig. 9-5. Three roller platform for stationary cycling on regular bicycle.

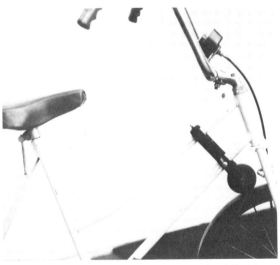

Fig. 9-6. Resistance is provided by roller wheel that turns against the cycle wheel.

228

caliper brakes that are adjustable to desired resistance against the bicycle rim, and a brake band that works over a heavy *flywheel*. Some inexpensive models have a brake band at the crank axle.

RECONDITIONING

Figure 9-7 shows a manufactured stationary exercise pedal cycle that I purchased in very poor condition at a junk store and reconditioned. I paid $10 for it. To recondition the cycle, I first disassembled it. The basic frame and stand was sanded and painted. New leg caps were added. The bottom bracket, pedals, and front hub (which has the sprocket) assemblies were overhauled, using the same techniques as for regular bicycles, as detailed previously. The chain and resistance wheel were cleaned and lubricated and the speedometer cable, which was broken, replaced. The result was an exercise bicycle in good condition for very little money and very little work on my part. This method is far easier

than building your own from used bicycle components, as detailed below. Where I live, I have seen a number of other similar used exercise bicycles suitable for reconditioning and some even in good working condition for low or at least reasonable prices. Secondhand and thrift stores, garage sales, and classified ads in local newspapers are good sources.

BUILDING EXERCISE CYCLES FROM BICYCLE COMPONENTS

I built the stationary exercise pedal cycle shown in Fig. 9-8 from inexpensive used bicycle parts. An old, damaged bicycle provided the bulk of the materials. Construction of the stand can vary considerably, as can the parts used in the construction. I used an inflated tire, but the smoothness of the ride is usually improved by using a solid tire. The wheel on mine is freewheeling with a coaster brake, but you might want to use a fixed wheel sprocket like those on track racing bicycles. The exact dimensions are not critical,

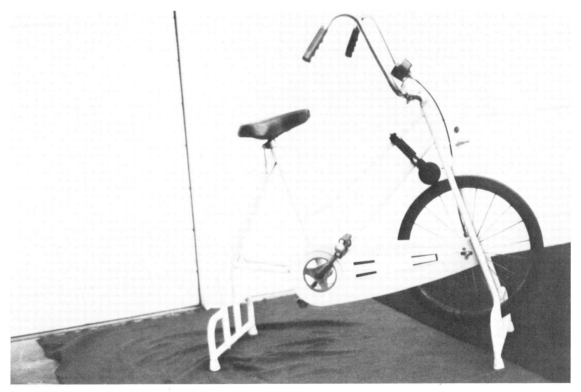

Fig. 9-7. Reconditioned stationary exercise cycle.

229

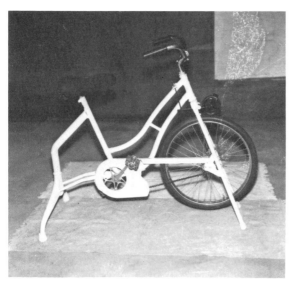

Fig. 9-8. Stationary exercise cycle constructed from bicycle parts.

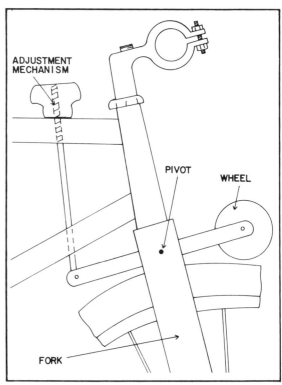

Fig. 9-9. Resistance wheel is pivot-mounted with adjusting bolt.

but it is important that the stand be sturdy. The base must be large enough so that the cycle will not tip and high enough to give ample clearance between pedals and ground at low points in the pedal cycles. The main section of the frame was taken from a regular bicycle. The front fork was brazed to the head tube so that the fork will not turn in the frame. The fork prongs are extended to form the stand.

The rear wheel, which becomes the front wheel on the exercise cycle, is mounted so that the chain tension can be adjusted. The mounts on the cycle shown were made from rear drop-outs cut from a bicycle frame, but you can also make these from flat steel material.

The resistance wheel (Fig. 9-9) is pivot-mounted with an adjusting bolt. The small wheel should be lined up with the cycle wheel. The arrangement shown allows hand adjustment of the resistance while you are exercising. Alternate resistance wheel possibilities include using a caliper brake (Fig. 9-10) assembly with a means of holding it to desired resistances against the rim and using a heavy flywheel (Fig. 9-11) in place of the bicycle wheel and an adjustable resistance or brake band.

The exercise cycle should have a chain guard. I made the one shown from a regular chain guard, reversed, and then added an angle iron extension by brazing it to the chain guard. Any type of chain guard that will keep clothing from getting caught between the chain and chainwheel and keep your clothing and skin from contacting the chain will suffice.

The construction of the exercise cycle shown requires brazing and/or welding. If you do not have the tools or skill to do this work yourself, you can have the brazing or welding done quite reasonably at a commercial shop, provided that you have everything ready—parts shaped, fitted, and even mounted in a jig—so that only the welding need be done.

Remember, most commercial firms charge by the hour or the amount of work they do, so it is to your advantage to make this as little as possible.

For the cycle shown, you will need to gather up the parts and materials. The best places that I've found for buying used bicycle frames and

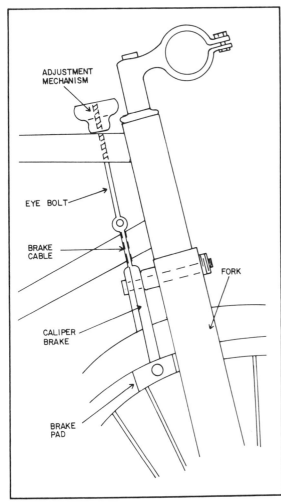

ADJUSTMENT
MECHANISM

EYE BOLT

BRAKE
CABLE

FORK

CALIPER
BRAKE

BRAKE
PAD

Fig. 9-10. Caliper brake used to provide resistance.

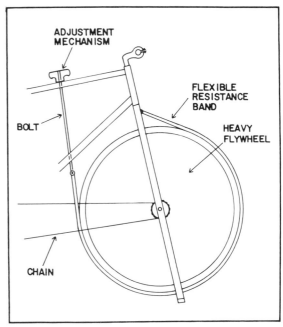

ADJUSTMENT
MECHANISM

BOLT

FLEXIBLE
RESISTANCE
BAND

HEAVY
FLYWHEEL

CHAIN

Fig. 9-11. Use of heavy flywheel and resistance brake band.

parts are city and county dumps that have sales yards. Other good sources include thrift and secondhand stores and garage sales.

As a rule, I suggest that you stick to standard steel frames and parts for building exercise pedal cycles. Aluminum alloy should be avoided where welding or brazing is required, as this material requires special equipment and know-how, and even then the joints might be inadequate.

In addition to the basic bicycle mechanics detailed above, you will also need to cut and shape bicycle frames and other components. For cutting bicycle frames, a hacksaw can be used. Whenever possible, fasten the frame in the padded jaws of a vise so that it is held firmly, and you can concentrate on the sawing. A tube cutter can be used to make perpendicular cuts on round tubing. This gives a neater cut than is possible with a hacksaw.

Bicycle frame tubing and similar tubing can be flattened in the jaws of a vise, although the degree to which this can be done without fracturing the tubing depends on the particular tubing and other factors.

Bent tubing, such as bicycle fork prongs, can often be straightened without heat by clamping the tubing between blocks of wood in a vise with the curved portion extending outward. A section of pipe that will just fit over the tubing is then used to gain leverage for straightening the tubing. Work carefully and readjust the position of the tubing in the vise as necessary. Try to avoid denting the tubing, because it will greatly weaken it.

Holes can be drilled in metal with a portable electric hand drill or a bench drill press and metal bits. A power bench grinder is useful for shaping bicycle frame sections and other grinding work. Hand files can also be used.

After you have the brazing and welding

done, you will probably want to smooth up the joints by grinding, filing, and sanding. The basic frame and stand is then painted. The bottom bracket, wheel assembly, chain, and other parts can be assembled. Add leg caps to the stand and handlebar grips to complete the construction.

OTHER STATIONARY PEDAL DEVICES

I purchased the pedal device with an adjustable brake resistance shown in Fig. 9-12 used at a secondhand store. I'm not exactly certain what its original intended use was. Perhaps it was designed for attachment to a hospital bed for reclining pedal exercise. In any case, I attached this device to a chair, as shown for sitting pedal exercise. This device could also be attached to a bench for reclined exercising.

Many years ago, I also constructed resistance pedal cycles for sitting and supine exercise, although these were intended mainly for laboratory experiments so that heart sounds, pulse waves, and other measurements could be taken while exercising with minimum upper body movement. These cycles do have possibilities as exercise machines, however.

While many stationary exercise devices have adjustable resistance, most do not tell you exactly what this resistance is (in foot-pounds or kilogram-meters, for example). To construct a resistance pedal cycle that does is much more difficult, and usually unnecessary for ordinary exercise and physical fitness riding. This becomes quite important for physical fitness and performance testing, however.

For home exercise use, it's being able to adjust the resistance that is important. It is also

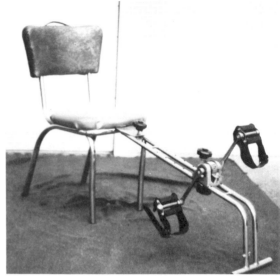

Fig. 9-12. Stationary resistance pedal device clamped to chair.

useful if there is a gauge or scale so that you will be able to set relative workloads and return to or progressively increase them.

A speedometer, which measures miles or kilometers per hour, and a mileage indicator are also useful devices. A timer can be used to control the length of the exercise period. A bell timer is useful here. Some manufactured stationary exercise bicycles have these as part of the cycles, but you can also use the household type, which are inexpensive and will serve essentially the same purpose.

Devices for monitoring heart rate are also available, some with feedback for changing the resistance of the workload to automatically keep the heart rate at a constant level.

Index